Blood

Blood:

The River of Life

By Jake Page
and the Editors of U.S.News Books

U.S.NEWS BOOKS Washington, D.C.

U.S.NEWS BOOKS

THE HUMAN BODY
Blood:
The River of Life

Editor/Publisher: Roy B. Pinchot

Series Editor: Judith Gersten

Contributing Editor: Linda S. Glisson

Picture Editor: Leah Bendavid-Val

Book Design: David M. Seager

Art Director: Jack Lanza

Art Coordinators
Irwin Glusker, Kristen Reilly

Staff Writers
Christopher West Davis,
Kathy E. Goldberg, Karen Jensen,
Michael Kitch, Charles R. Miller,
Doug M. Podolsky, Matthew J. Schudel,
Robert D. Selim, Edward O. Welles, Jr.

Director of Text Research: William Rust

Chief Researcher: Bruce A. Lewenstein

Text Researchers
Allison Abood, Susana Barañano,
Barbara L. Buchman, Heléne Goldberg,
Michael C. McCarthy, E. Cameron
Ritchie, Loraine S. Suskind,

Picture Researchers
Jean Shapiro Cantú, Gregg Johnson,
Ronald M. Davis, Leora Kahn,
Chandley McDonald, David Ross,
Lynn Russillo

Technical Illustration Layout
Esperance Shatarah

Art Staff
Raymond J. Ferry, Martha Anne Scheele

Director of Production: Harold F. Chevalie

Production Coordinator: Diane B. Freed

Production Assistant: Mary Ann Haas

Production Staff
Carol Bashara, Ina Bloomberg,
Barbara M. Clark, Glenna Mickelson,
Sharon Turner

Quality Control Director: Joseph Postilion

Director of Sales: James Brady

Business Planning: Robert Licht

Fulfillment Director: Debra Hasday Fanshel

Fulfillment Assistant: Diane Childress

Cover Design: Moonink Communications

Cover Art: Paul Giovanopoulos

Author

Jake Page is a contributing editor to *Science 82*
and author of the column "Jake's Page."
Formerly an editor of *Smithsonian* magazine
and publisher of Smithsonian Exposition
Books, Mr. Page has also contributed to
other magazines, including *National Geographic,*
Horticulture and *American Film.*

Series Consultants

Donald M. Engelman is Molecular Biophysicist and Biochemist at Yale University and a
guest Biophysicist at the Brookhaven National
Laboratory in New York. A specialist in biological structure, Dr. Engelman has published
research in American and European journals.
From 1976 to 1980, he was chairman of the
Molecular Biology Study Section at the
National Institutes of Health.

Stanley Joel Reiser is Associate Professor of
Medical History at Harvard Medical School
and codirector of the Kennedy Interfaculty
Program in Medical Ethics at the University.
He is the author of *Medicine and the Reign of
Technology* and coeditor of *Ethics in Medicine:
Historical Perspectives and Contemporary Concerns.*

Harold C. Slavkin, Professor of Biochemistry
at the University of Southern California,
directs the Graduate Program in Craniofacial
Biology and also serves as Chief of the
Laboratory for Developmental Biology in the
University's Gerontology Center. His research
on the genetic basis of congenital defects of
the head and neck has been widely published.

Lewis Thomas is Chancellor of the Memorial
Sloan-Kettering Cancer Center in New York
City. A member of the National Academy of
Sciences, Dr. Thomas has served on advisory
councils of the National Institutes of Health.
He has written *The Medusa and the Snail* and
The Lives of a Cell, which received the 1974
National Book Award in Arts and Letters.

Consultants for Blood

Robert A. Good, head of the Cancer Research
Program at the Oklahoma Medical Research
Foundation, has contributed significantly to
the understanding of the mechanisms of
immunity. Formerly President and Director of
the Sloan-Kettering Institute for Cancer
Research, Dr. Good received the Albert Lasker
Clinical Medical Research Award in 1970 for
his contributions to the fields of immunology
and cellular engineering. He has written many
medical books and authored more than 1,500
articles for scientific journals.

Lawrence S. Lessin is Director of the Division
of Hematology and Oncology at the George
Washington University Medical Center in
Washington, D.C. He is currently conducting
a six-year research study on sickle cell anemia.
Dr. Lessin also contributes to a variety of
scientific journals, including *Nature, Annals of
Internal Medicine* and *Blood,* the journal of the
American Society of Hematology.

Kenneth C. Robbins is Scientific Director of
the Michael Reese Research Foundation, a
large research and blood center in Chicago. He
is a member of the International Committee
on Thrombosis and Hemostasis. He is also
Professor of Medicine and Pathology at the
University of Chicago's Pritzker School of
Medicine. Dr. Robbins received the *Prix
Servier* Medal from the *Institut de Recherche
Servier* in 1980 for his outstanding achievements in the field of fibrinolysis. He has
authored many articles on the fibrinolytic
mechanisms of blood, beginning with his discovery of the fibrin-stabilizing factor in 1944.

Picture Consultants

Amram Cohen is General Surgery Resident at
the Walter Reed Army Medical Center in
Washington, D.C.

Richard G. Kessel, Professor of Zoology at
the University of Iowa, studies cells, tissues
and organs with scanning and transmission
electron microscopy instruments. He is
coauthor of two books on electron microscopy.

**U.S.News Books, a division of
U.S.News & World Report, Inc.**

**Library of Congress
Cataloging in Publication Data**

Page, Jake.
  Blood, the river of life.

  (The Human body)
  Includes indexes.
  1. Blood. 2. Blood — Diseases. I. U.S.
News Books. II. Title. III. Series.
QP91.P25   612'.11   81–16323
                                 AACR2
ISBN 0–89193–604–1
ISBN 0–89193–634–3 (Leatherbound)
ISBN 0–89193–664–5 (School ed.)

20 19 18 17 16 15 14 13 12 11
10   9   8   7   6   5   4   3   2   1

Contents

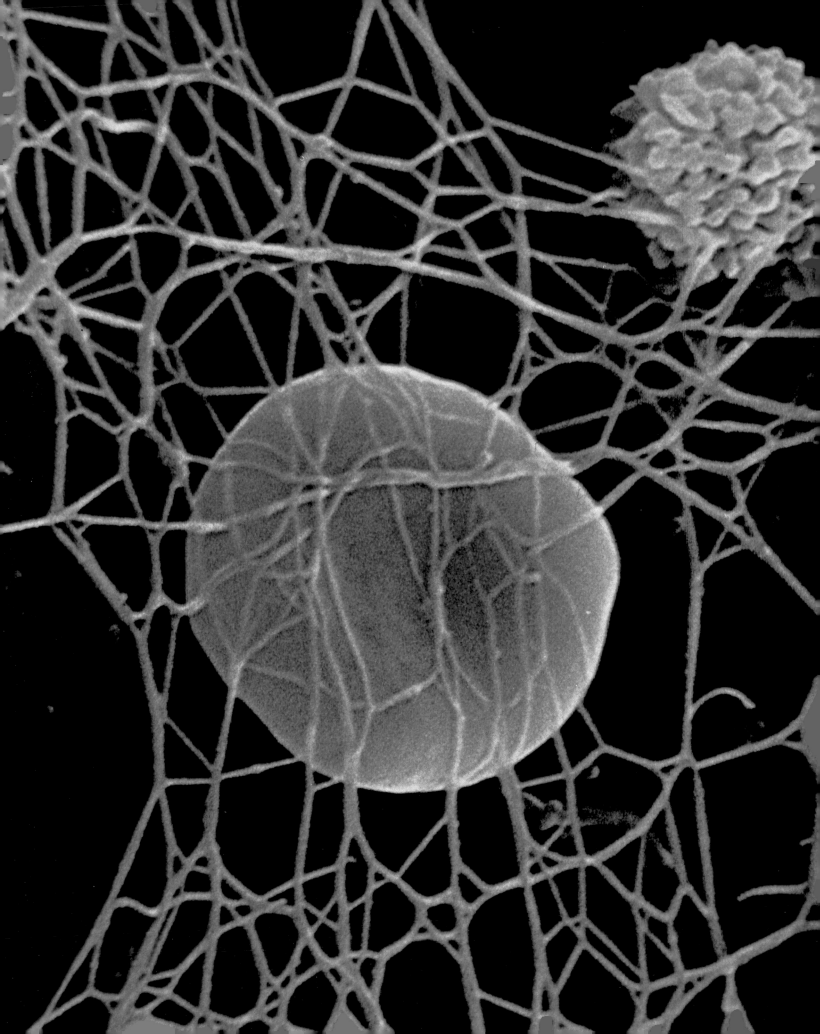

Introduction:

The Magical Current

Blood is a liquid tissue, a complex potion whose every design expresses the magic of life. At its figurative center — the iron in the tissue's soul — lie the predominant red blood cells. They give blood its familiar color and endow it with its functional essence. Carrying vital oxygen to the other tissues, red blood cells course through a sea rich in hormones, vitamins, proteins and enzymes. This is the chemical ebb and flow of blood, the restless tidal shifts that assure the body's delicate internal balance.

Through this teeming array there flow deeper currents, the blood's healing instincts, its urge to instantly seal and mend the slightest of wounds. This impulse to clot — to conserve — affirms the tissue's basic nature. It is an essence, a substance more potent than its modest measure. In the five-and-a-half quarts of blood in the adult human body lies an arrangement of cells which safeguard survival in a world of microbial hazard. These white cells, about one-tenth of 1 percent of the blood, hold the power to detect, identify and destroy millions of deadly microorganisms. By his blood, man builds a barrier more formidable than the highest wall. The blood is a potent reminder of man's biological success, his will as a species to survive.

It, too, is a tie through time, a symbolic link between man's mythic past and his modern present. Through blood flows the same mineral balance as that of the seas of the Cambrian era, half a billion years ago. From this primordial ocean, it is thought, life first emerged to exist on land. Today, scientists peering into the blood's shifting currents now see patterns that enable the early detection of many diseases. Ultimately, blood unites not only the ages but emotion and experience, too. Long the object of ceremony and myth, blood stirs a wealth of passions from hope to fear. From blood, symbol of man's mortality, springs the unending river of life.

Under a scanning electron microscope's silvery light, threads of fibrin, a clotting agent, spin a cocoon around the shimmering world of a single red blood cell. By such deft design, fibrin conveys the blood's innate urge to preserve itself — and therefore life.

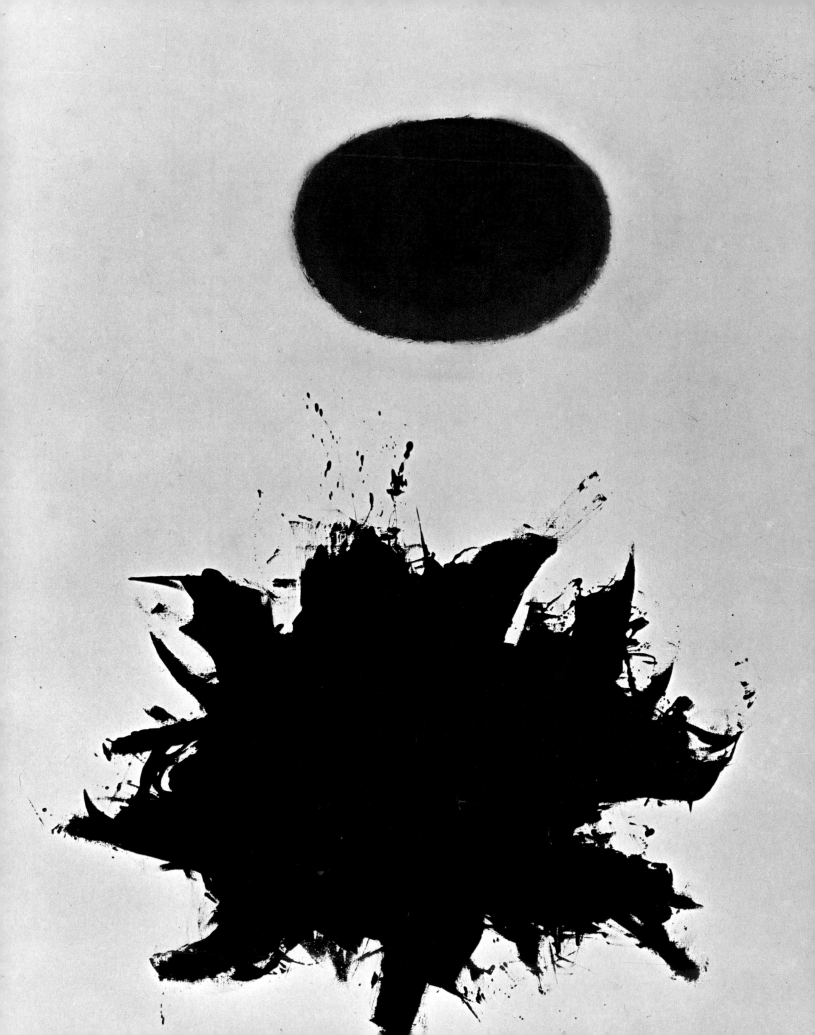

Chapter 1

A Living Symbol

Traditions passed down from the earliest days of mankind have equated blood with the energy of life, the source of courage and health. Blood's quiet, pulsing strength made it a symbol of powers that controlled the destiny of every living thing. For primitive man, the world was full of incomprehensible forces. Winds blew and brought sudden rain; the sun might shine relentlessly, bringing drought and famine; disease could silently strike down entire settlements; and once-invincible warriors were felled by enemies or enfeebled by advancing age. Early societies frequently devised elaborate systems of belief to give meaning to what happened around them. The natural world and superstition merged as man strove to order his universe.

When hunters speared an animal, they could see its blood flow from the wound. When it ceased, the animal was dead. A simple necessity, the gathering of food, quickly became bound up with faith, philosophy and mystery. In some cultures, people drank blood to gain strength from the life-giving fluid. When a warrior of ancient Scythia killed his first opponent in battle, he drank his victim's blood to acquire courage. Blood rites have remained an important part of cultural identity into modern times.

To the Masai tribe of Kenya and Tanzania, blood figures prominently as both an everyday item and an object of ceremony. With arrows inserted quickly and painlessly into the necks of cattle, the Masai withdraw blood for food. It is drunk either fresh or mixed with milk and forms a supplementary part of their diet in times of drought or nomadic migration. The Masai hold the lion in a place of honor. For a man to assume a lion's fabled strength and courage, he must drink its blood. Blood also measures in their system of justice. If a tribal member has been accused of cattle stealing, he must drink blood and recite, "If I have stolen the cattle this blood will

Soaring above chaotic blackness, a crimson droplet radiates with its own vibrant energy. Associated with blood throughout history, the color red is a symbol of brilliance, health, the sustaining hope of life.

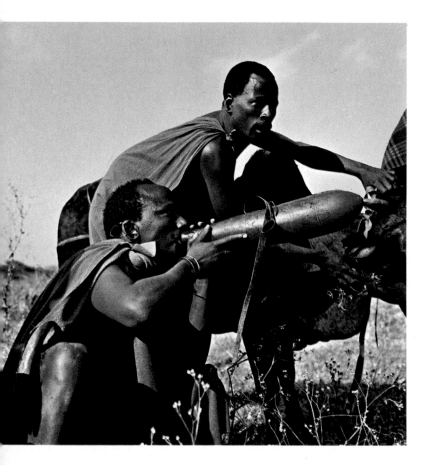

In the desolate savanna of the Great Rift Valley in Kenya and Tanzania, members of the Masai tribe routinely supplement their diet with cow's blood. Drawn painlessly from the jugular veins of cattle, the blood is often mixed with milk in a hollow gourd and drunk during times when food is scarce.

kill me." Presumably, he dies within two weeks if guilty and survives unharmed if innocent.

Orthodox Jews, however, scrupulously avoid the partaking of blood, as directed by scripture. Before being labeled kosher, carcasses must be drained of blood before a butcher dresses them. Until recently, the Roman Catholic Church forbade the eating of red meat on Fridays.

Regeneration and Renewal

Whether its presence is actual or symbolic, blood has long been associated with food and drink. The bacchanals of classical times were not binges of unfettered revelry. Rooted in solemn rites of fertility and regeneration, Dionysus (or Bacchus, as he was known to the Romans) symbolized the steady motion of blood through the body. As god of the vine, he represented the sap of life, the surging excitement and renewal of nature. To the Greeks, wine was both the bountiful produce of Dionysus and a sacrament to him. Wine represented his blood, his vital element. Drinking wine elevated mortal man, to make him more godlike, possessed of a power greater than himself. Dionysian rites transcended even the act of homage to a god: they were taken to be the actual sharing of his divinity through the drinking of blood-colored wine.

Current throughout the Biblical era, the legend of Dionysus parallels later religious feasts of celebration. According to Jewish tradition, God warned Moses that the angel of death would claim the first-born son of every family as the final plague on Egypt. To avoid the catastrophe, Jewish families were to spread the blood of a lamb on their doorposts as a sign to the angel that he should pass over their houses. Moses then led the exodus of the Israelites out of Egypt. Modern-day Jews commemorate this salvation each spring during Passover. A Passover feast, the Seder, celebrates the delivery from Egypt.

The Seder took on significance to Christians because it was during one such feast that Christ last appeared together with the apostles, in what is now known as the Last Supper. Surrounded by his disciples, Christ passed a cup of wine among them, with each of the twelve taking a sip: "And he said unto them, This is my blood of the new

Riotous festivals in classical times honored Dionysus, god of the vine. French painter Nicolas Poussin depicts revelers celebrating the powers of wine, symbolic of the blood of Dionysus and the spirit of life.

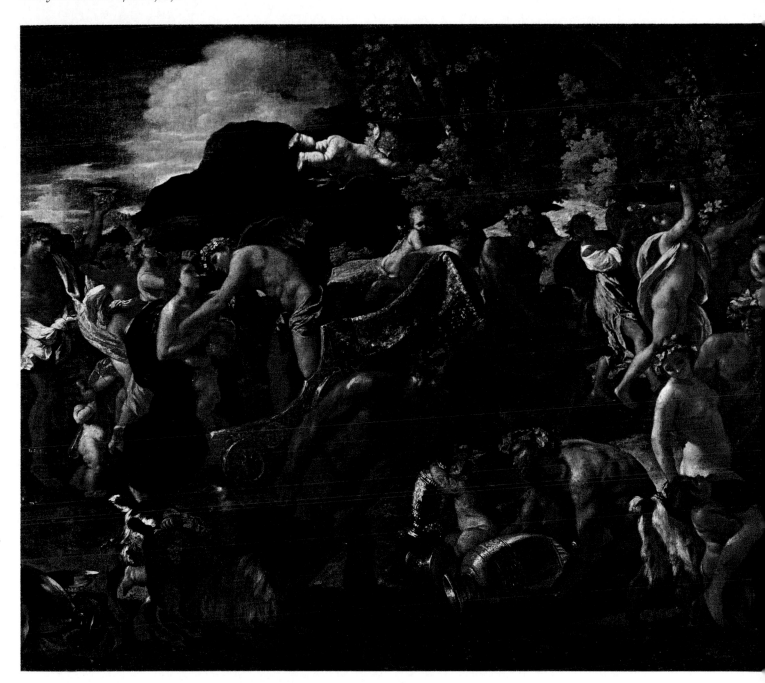

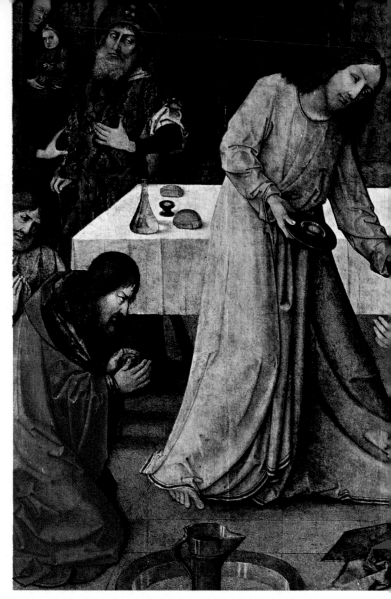

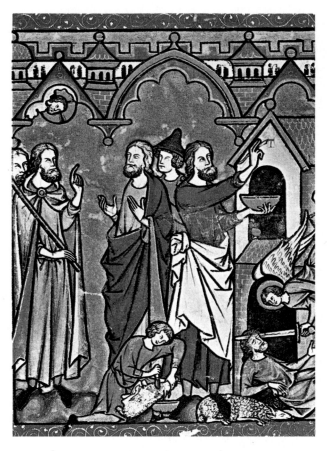

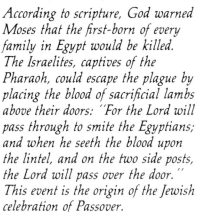

According to scripture, God warned Moses that the first-born of every family in Egypt would be killed. The Israelites, captives of the Pharaoh, could escape the plague by placing the blood of sacrificial lambs above their doors: "For the Lord will pass through to smite the Egyptians; and when he seeth the blood upon the lintel, and on the two side posts, the Lord will pass over the door." This event is the origin of the Jewish celebration of Passover.

testament, which is shed for many." The most solemn Christian rite, Communion re-creates the Last Supper with the symbolic drinking of Christ's blood. Some believe that by the act of transubstantiation Eucharistic wine becomes literally the blood of Christ.

A baffling phenomenon in Naples, Italy, held to be a miracle by the Catholic Church, has puzzled scientists and clergy alike for centuries. Eighteen times a year, at predictable intervals, the dried blood of St. Januarius suddenly liquefies. Scientists are skeptical of the phenomenon because it was not reported until the fourteenth century, more than a thousand years after the saint's death. Besides, under normal circumstances, blood cannot return to a liquid state once it has congealed and dried. They have examined the hermetically sealed glass reliquary in which the blood is kept but cannot account for the blood's periodic transformation.

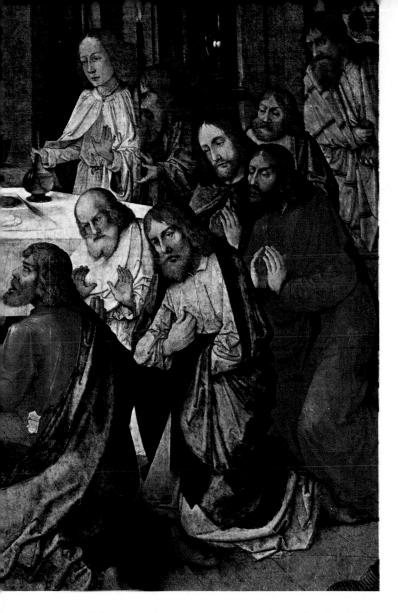

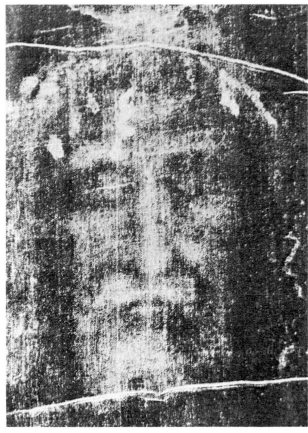

Mentioned more than 500 times in the Bible, blood becomes a promise of atonement to believers through covenants, or agreements, with God. Christ's shedding of blood at the Crucifixion represents the hope of salvation. For many people, the term "blood of Christ" signifies more than metaphor. The mysterious shroud of Turin, said to have been placed over Christ's body after the Crucifixion, shows, in reversed patterns like a photographic negative, the outline of a man resembling traditional portrayals of Jesus. Traces of blood from wounds described in Biblical accounts are visible, the head is crowned with thorns, and coins rest on the eyelids — a common practice at the time of Christ. Scientists performing sophisticated tests on the fragile shroud have concluded that it is not a forgery and that it dates from the Crucifixion era. There is no way of proving, though, that the image on the shroud is indeed that of Christ.

At the Last Supper, above left, Christ offered his disciples bread and wine as sacramental tokens of his flesh and blood. The shroud of Turin, above right, is believed by many to be the cloth that covered Christ after his death. The well-preserved fabric dates from the time of Christ, bears the image of a bearded man and is stained with blood from wounds similar to those described in New Testament accounts of the Crucifixion.

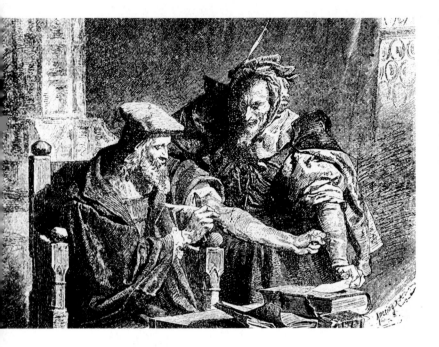

More elusive than the tale of the shroud is the legend of the Holy Grail. The object of quest by knights throughout the Middle Ages, the Grail was considered the chalice of the Last Supper and was thought to contain the blood of Christ.

An Inviolate Bond

Blood can also, through diabolical intervention, be an agent of doom. The Faust legend, dating from the Middle Ages, takes its force from a pact with the devil that Faust signs with his own blood. In Christopher Marlowe's play of 1592, Doctor Faustus, as he is called, writes in blood from his own arm, sealing his fate:

> Lo, Mephistophilis, for love of thee,
> I cut mine arm, and with my proper blood
> Assure my soul to be great Lucifer's,
> Chief lord and regent of perpetual night.

Pacts with the devil may be the stuff of drama and folklore, but alliances between individuals have long been secured with the mingling of blood. In societies where blood brotherhood exists, it is more inviolate than marriage. Blood brothers are bound to defend each other from attack and to avenge a wrongful act with death, if necessary. With these bonds of blood, an outsider can enter a clan with the full rights of kinship as though he were descended from the same ancestry. Blood brotherhood and similar forms of blood alliance exist throughout the world.

In many primitive cultures, the belief in blood sacrifice is still strong. The sacrifice, whether of people or animals, is looked upon as a duty to the gods. The purpose of the sacrifice is to make an offering of blood, not flesh, since only blood has the power to renew life. Until the last century some American Indian tribes sacrificed a young man or woman at the beginning of each planting season to ensure plentiful crops. A few drops of blood were sprinkled over the seeds to give them added potency. In parts of Africa, Asia and South America, natives ceremoniously sacrifice animals to increase the fertility of their plants and to appease their gods. In both ancient and modern times, drinking the blood of sacrificial animals was believed to confer oracular powers.

In ancient Phrygia young communicants underwent an unusual blood ritual to affirm their devotion to the god Attis. According to the myth, Attis was a handsome youth, the favorite of Cybele, the principal goddess in the Phrygian pantheon. Because Attis loved another, however, Cybele placed a curse on him that drove him mad. Under this spell Attis castrated himself and died. Cybele repented and obtained a promise from Zeus that Attis's body would never decay. As a result, Attis came to symbolize resurrection.

To pay Attis full respect, a young man had to undergo a baptism of blood. Having fasted, he stood beneath a wooden grate onto which a garlanded bull was led. With a consecrated spear, priests killed the bull, letting its blood run through the grate onto the worshiper below, who bathed himself in the blood and emerged scarlet from the pit. By washing away his sins in the blood of the bull, the follower of Attis had the hope of eternal life.

The primitive belief that blood is life itself, the animating force, survives in unexpected ways. Even in our own time, much misunderstanding persists about menstruation. Fear of menstrual blood originates in the superstitious notion that any blood expelled from the body contains evil spirits in conflict with the blood of life that stays

Among the bloodiest civilizations
in history, the Aztecs of Mexico
made human sacrifices to their gods.
Young people were sacrificed in
elaborate religious ceremonies
presided over by priests.

within the veins and arteries. Roman naturalist Pliny described menstruation as "a fatal poison, corrupting and decomposing urine, depriving seeds of their fecundity, destroying insects, blasting garden flowers and grasses, causing fruits to fall from branches [and] dulling razors." In the sixteenth century, noted Swiss physician Paracelsus maintained that the devil created all insects from menstrual blood.

Frequently, women are confined during menses, separated from the company of men and from normal activities. In parts of Asia and the South Pacific, girls at puberty must stay in bed or in isolated huts for weeks or months at a time. In certain societies of India, however, menarche is a more joyous occasion. Family members gather to wish the girl a fertile life and to celebrate the beginning of womanhood with a feast.

A Sorcery of Its Own

Legends frequently depict blood as a dangerous fluid capable of harming those who merely touch it. Until relatively recent times, there was a common English belief that land sullied by human blood was accursed and made barren. Today, in some regions of Africa, blood dripping to the ground must be carefully rubbed into the dirt to prevent witch doctors from using it in potions.

Through a kind of sorcery of its own, blood was long thought to reveal true feelings and so could unmask criminals. A corpse could identify its murderer. Even kings could be accused. When English king Richard the Lion-Hearted stood before the slain body of his father Henry II in 1189, blood was said to have flowed from Henry's nostrils. Although he did not murder Henry, Richard had been prepared to overthrow his father.

Four hundred years later, philosopher and scholar Francis Bacon noted: "It is an usual observation that if the body of one murthered be brought before the murtherer, the wounds will bleed afresh." The superstition was used as legal evidence in 1688. A jury, having heard testimony that blood flowed from the body of Sir James Standsfield when touched by his son Philip, convicted Philip of murder.

For all the primitive worship of blood as a potent symbol of life, blood has come to represent

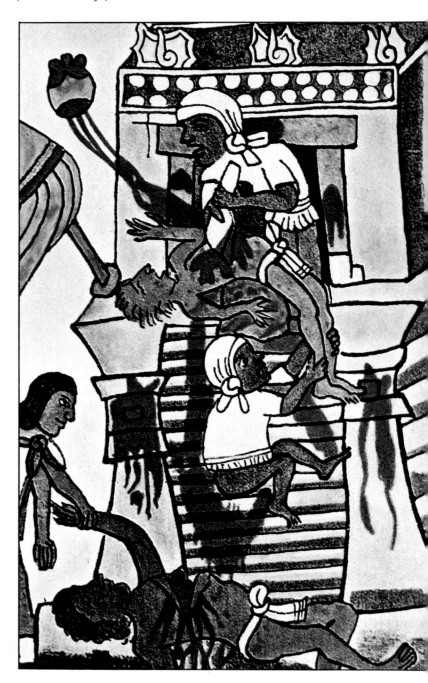

"The chase, the sport of kings;
Image of war, without its guilt,"
wrote poet William Somerville in
1735. Known as a "blood sport,"
fox hunting is rich in traditions that
have changed little in centuries.

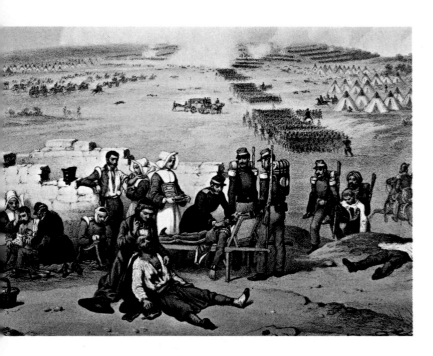

Many medical advances have taken
place on the battlefield, but the
toll of war has weighed heavily in
the conscience of mankind. War has
been seen both as a noble endeavor,
drawing on centuries-old traditions
of valor, and as sorrowful futility,
symbolized by needless bloodshed.

in modern Western societies the loss of life and the futility of war. The images of war are sometimes heroic and associated with high-minded, worthwhile causes. In this light, the shedding of blood is valorous, for its sacrifice is a noble ideal. "The tree of liberty," declared Thomas Jefferson, "must be refreshed from time to time with the blood of patriots and tyrants." Jefferson's view of war was not new. Thousands of years before, Greek poet Homer glorified the heroes of the Trojan War in the *Iliad*. Many passages equate death in battle with glory as blood spills onto the plains of Troy.

War, the Red Animal

But the American image of war changed dramatically during the Civil War. The number of deaths staggered citizens on both sides of the Mason-Dixon line. Stephen Crane epitomized this new ambiguity toward war in *The Red Badge of Courage*, published in 1895. Individual glory was tainted as the soldiers marched "to look at war, the red animal — war, the blood-swollen god." The unnamed soldier at the center of the story envied his wounded comrades: "He wished that he, too, had a wound, a red badge of courage."

World War I was the event that jolted the world from such innocence. Never before had blood flowed so freely for so long and for so little gain. The English were especially aware of the war's futility. Roses and poppies, flowers the color of blood, became part of the mythology of the First World War. "For ordinary people," writes literary scholar Paul Fussell, "roses connoted loyalty to England, service to it, and sacrifice to it." One sentimental anecdote tells of "a tall rose tree with crimson roses blooming even in autumn" that grew from the grave of an English sergeant who was killed while venturing out of the trenches toward no man's land on Christmas Day, 1915. British military cemeteries in France are still decorated with roses.

The flower most readily associated with World War I is the poppy. In both England and the United States poppies made of paper are sometimes worn to commemorate the soldiers and battles. The California poppy, most common in America, is orange or yellow. But the European

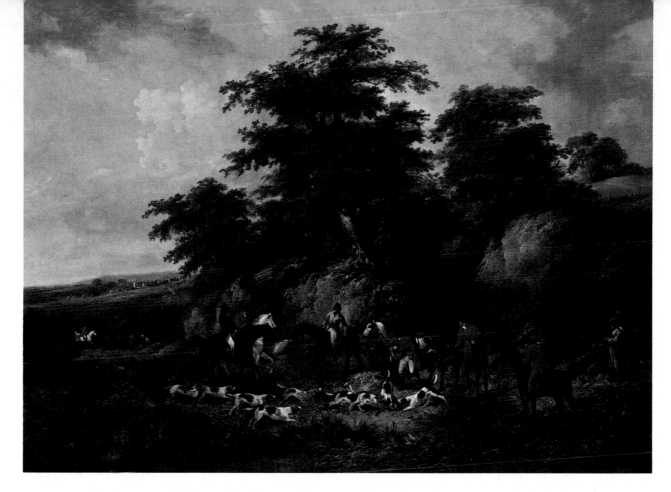

poppy is a brilliant scarlet. It is this poppy that, in the words of a popular British poem of the era, grows "In Flanders fields . . . Between the crosses, row on row," nourished, according to legend, by the blood of fallen soldiers.

If the British have become disillusioned with the hopelessness of war, they still maintain an almost martial spirit in sport. Considered a leisurely pastime by some, an embarrassing anachronism by others, fox hunting has been a fixture of the English and American countrysides for centuries. Something of an enigma as a sport, fox hunting is both dignified and cruel, feeding on traditions whose origins are now obscured by time. Oscar Wilde, poking fun at the amusements of the English gentry, once quipped that fox hunting was "the unspeakable in full pursuit of the uneatable." A "blood sport" because, in the end, the fox is killed, fox hunting is a ritual reminiscent of pagan practices. At the conclusion of the hunt, the group leader daubs blood from the carcass onto the faces of new members of the hunting party. When novices are so "blooded," they are sometimes called "young bloods."

The language of blood expresses temperament, lineage and violence. The temperature of blood corresponds with events and the emotions they inspire in "blood-chilling," "bloodcurdling," and "to make one's blood boil." When we say someone is "hot-blooded," we mean that he has little control over his emotions, is excitable and has a ready temper. Conversely, a cold-blooded person is rational and controlled. Thus, to murder "in cold blood" is doubly heinous because the crime has been rationally planned. Today, the term "blood bath" evokes the horror of slaughter, but in ancient Egypt it was a medical treatment for leprosy and elephantiasis, a lymphatic disorder causing swollen limbs. Hebraic records give a grisly account of the practice: "When the leprous Pharaohs were advised by their astrologers to bathe in human blood, they commanded the slaughter of 150 Jewish children every morning and evening." Spanish aristocrats of Castile originated the term "blue blood" to set themselves apart from the darker-skinned Spaniards of Moorish descent. The nobles' light skin revealed veins carrying bluish-looking blood. In time, any well-born Spaniard could claim to have blue blood. "Bad blood" between people suggests ill will, particularly of a long-standing feud. The expression comes from medieval notions of physiology, when it was thought that external forces could alter the character of the blood.

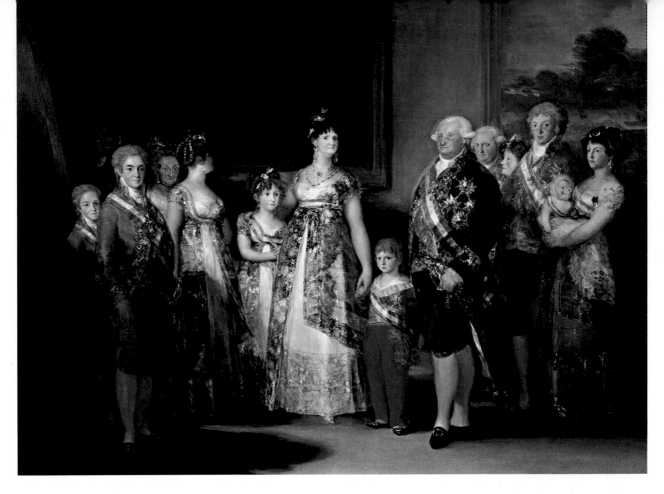

The royal family of Charles IV, King of Spain, posed for Francisco Goya in 1800. Descended from long lines of aristocratic ancestors, Spanish rulers claimed to have sangre azul, *blue blood. The tradition of blue blood originated when Castilian nobles noticed the bluish veins under their pale skin. Their darker-skinned subjects could not see their veins so easily and thus could not boast of a distinguished heritage.*

The color red has taken on considerable symbolic meaning from its association with blood. In early cultures, every red substance could be a surrogate of blood. In Chinese tomb art, noblemen were often portrayed in red to give the promise of everlasting health. In ancient Rome, generals rode through the streets with their faces colored red to show they were courageous and victorious in war. Frequently associated with happiness and good health, red has often been considered a healing color. Red coral and carnelian jewelry has been worn to stimulate the life-giving power of blood. Novelist Sir Walter Scott made broad medicinal claims for bloodstone, a red-flecked, dark green semiprecious stone. In *The Talisman,* Scott asserted that bloodstone "stauncheth blood, driveth away poison, preserveth health; Yea, some maintain that it provoketh rain and darkeneth the sun, suffering not him that beareth it to be abused." The ruby, traditionally linked to Mars, the god of war, is sometimes taken as a symbol of war's spirit of violence and destruction.

Blood was a symbol of life and strength long before ancient physicians were able to explore its properties and follow its passage through the body. The earliest records on the physiology of

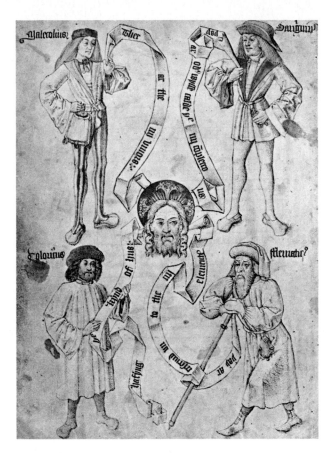

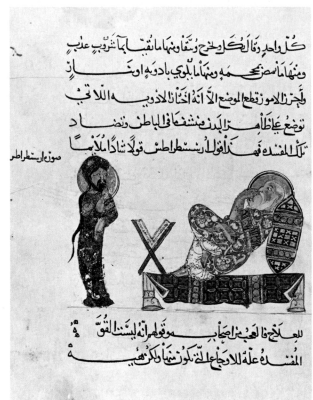

Blood was often thought to have curative powers in the Middle Ages, particularly when combined with magic. With sympathetic healing, a common practice in Europe, illness or pain was believed to travel to an external substance that would take on the illness. The "sympathetic" substitute could then be treated to cure the patient. From such a premise, the sympathetic egg was born. A chicken egg, drained and refilled with warm human blood, was carefully sealed and placed under a brooding hen. Next, it was cooked in an oven for several hours. Finally, it was placed over a patient's wound or pain. When the illness was thought to have left the patient's body to be absorbed in the blood-filled egg, the egg was taken away and buried.

Another form of sympathetic healing, practiced throughout the Middle Ages and as late as the seventeenth century in the British Isles, treated wounds by applying green vitriol to blood from a wound. Green vitriol, better known today as iron sulfate, could also heal a wound when applied to a bloodstained cloth taken from an injured soldier or duelist. As long as the garment was rubbed with the solution, the patient was expected to recover, regardless of how far away he might be.

The belief that the body consisted of four elements, or humors, governing the moods of man endured from the time of ancient Greeks until the Renaissance. An illustration in the guild book of the barber-surgeons of York, dating from about 1500, shows, clockwise from upper left, melancholy, sanguine, phlegmatic and choleric humors. Blood was associated with the sanguine humor, most desirable of the four. Among the first to challenge the theory of the four humors with experimental evidence was Erasistratus, the renowned physician of Alexandria, Egypt, in the third century B.C. He is shown above, reclining, in an illustration from a thirteenth-century Arabic medical manuscript.

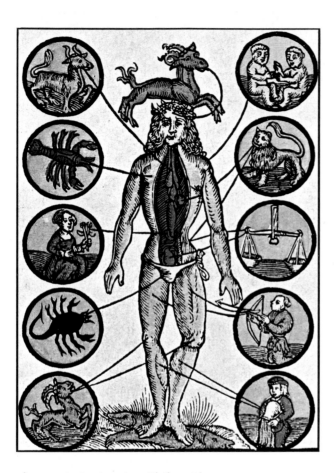

A common treatment until the mid-1800s, bloodletting was performed under a variety of scientific and superstitious rituals. This German woodcut from 1512 related various parts of the body to the signs of the zodiac. Bloodletting was considered most effective during April, May and September.

Bloodletting, the deliberate removal of small amounts of blood from the body, is an ancient treatment that originated with the Egyptian dynasties and survived until the nineteenth century. Pliny recorded that early physicians learned of bloodletting, or phlebotomy, from observing the hippopotamus. When the hippopotamus had overeaten, it would supposedly lower itself over a sharp reed and puncture a blood vessel. When enough blood had drained to make the animal comfortable, it would stop the wound by rubbing its belly in limey earth.

Medieval doctors developed elaborate methods for bleeding their patients, relying on astrological charts and religious sanction to get the most favorable results. Churches commonly had special rooms set aside for bloodletting. Many treatises from the Middle Ages, some in verse, prescribed regimens for bloodletting and ethical codes for physicians. Doctors were advised to be courteous to their patients and to make shallow incisions when withdrawing blood "so that from sinewes you all hurt do keepe." Prescriptions often contained complete recipes as well as gentle reminders on drinking, cleanliness and general behavior. A thirteenth-century Latin manuscript translated into English verse in 1608 described the expected benefits of bloodletting:

> By bleeding, to the marrow commeth heat,
> It maketh cleane your braine, relieves your
>   eye,
> It mends your appetite, restoreth sleepe,
> Correcting humours that do waking keepe:
> All inward parts and senses also clearing,
> It mends the voyce, touch, smell & tast, &
>   hearing.

The foremost physician in the early days of American independence, Benjamin Rush, strongly advocated bloodletting as a remedy for many ailments. Phlebotomy had long since become a panacea, often applied recklessly. In December of 1799, when George Washington's throat was swollen tight by excess fluids, his physicians drew so much blood from him that he had no strength to fight the infection. The illness might have been fatal anyway, but one of the general's attending physicians later wrote that if they had

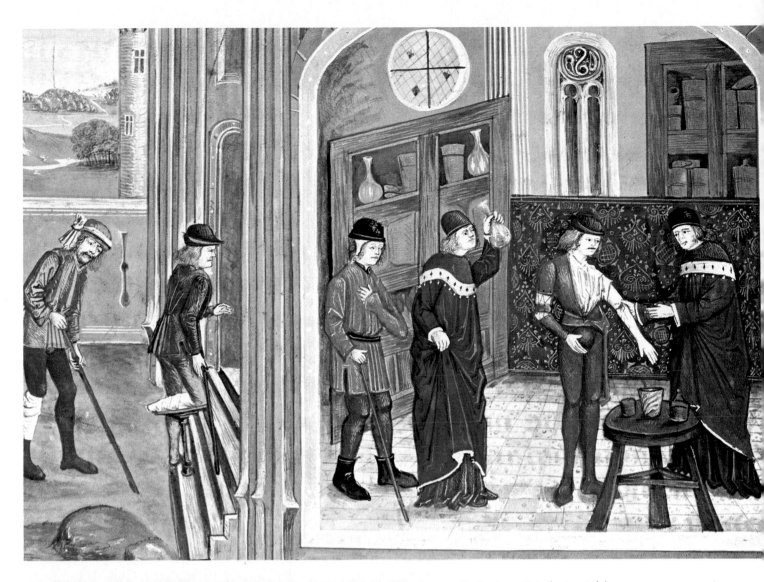

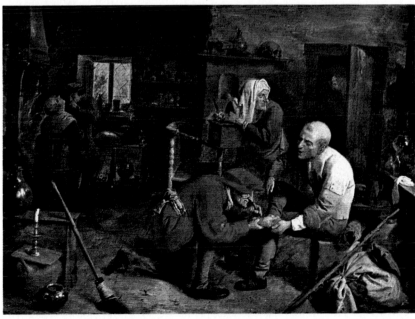

Patients wait to be treated by medieval physicians, above. This fifteenth-century French illustration depicts two of the most common medical practices of the time — bloodletting and urine analysis. As an adjunct to their profession, barbers performed many kinds of surgery, including bloodletting. Shown in a Flemish painting from about 1630, left, barbers often saw their patients in crowded and dirty rooms. Drawing blood from the feet was a standard practice.

A sixteenth-century barber-surgeon,
Ambroise Paré pioneered a number
of advances in surgery. As field
doctor to the French army, he developed safe methods for treating
wounds and controlling bleeding.

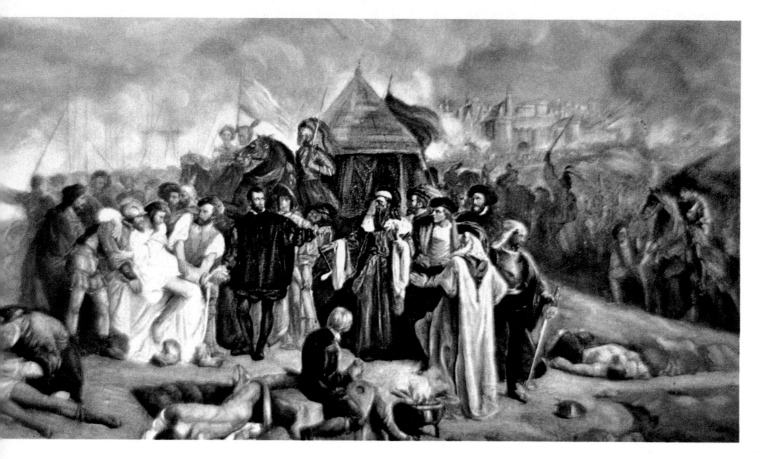

"taken no more blood from him, our good friend might have been alive now." It is still possible in some parts of Europe and the United States to buy leeches for drawing off blood, but phlebotomy has not been widely used as a serious medical treatment since the mid-nineteenth century. Nevertheless, when Joseph Stalin lay dying from a stroke in 1953, Soviet doctors applied leeches in a futile effort to save his life.

Until relatively recent times, bloodletting and surgery were considered forms of manual labor and thus were not worthy pursuits of gentlemen. By the end of the eleventh century, this custom had created an entire subprofessional class — the barber-surgeon. Under ecclesiastic law, monks of the Middle Ages had to be bled from time to time. Because barbers made regular circuits to clip the monks' tonsures, they eventually began to perform the bloodletting as well. In cities and villages, barbers placed white cloths, red with

blood, outside their doors to indicate the most efficacious times for bleeding. This early mode of advertisement survives today in the form of familiar red and white spiral-striped barber poles.

Ambroise Paré, trained as a barber-surgeon, and a field surgeon to the French army in the sixteenth century, was a man of no formal education, but he nonetheless was familiar with the works of Galen and other physicians. At first, he followed most of the accepted practices of his time, including that of treating gunshot wounds with boiling oil. In 1536, though, during the siege of Turin, Paré ran out of oil. In an effort to stanch the soldiers' bleeding, he applied a mixture of egg yolk, oil of roses and turpentine to the wounds. To his surprise, he found that the wounds he had dressed with this mixture "were not inflamed nor tumefied; but on the contrary the others that were burnt with the scalding oil were feverish, tormented with much pain, and the parts about their wounds were swollen." For saving the lives of men wounded in battle, soldiers carried Paré through the streets on their shoulders. In 1545, he restored the ligature, a method of tying off bleeding vessels known in classical times, in favor of cauterizing wounds to sear the veins shut. After he retired from the wars, he was called to minister to the Duke d'Auret of Flanders, suffering from a gunshot wound in the leg. As part of the treatment, Paré prescribed flowers for the Duke's bedroom, a device that simulated the sound of rain, music "to lift the patient's spirit" and comedians "to make him merry."

Science Surfaces

Andreas Vesalius and Miguel Servetus, two young scholars of the sixteenth century, published works that challenged Galen's description of circulation. Vesalius's 663-page folio appeared in 1543. Leading medical authorities of the day attacked Vesalius harshly, eventually forcing him out of the University of Padua in Italy into an exile of oblivion in Spain. Servetus fared worse. He combined anatomical studies with theology and, in 1546, disproved the prevailing Galenic doctrine that blood passed through walls in the heart from one chamber to another. His scientific and religious views constituted a heretical mix, for which he was burned at the stake in 1553.

In seventeenth-century Jacobean England, William Harvey built on the ideas of Vesalius, Servetus and Italian physician Andrea Cesalpino to formulate his theory of blood circulation. He studied anatomy at Cambridge and the world-famous University of Padua before joining the court of James I as royal physician. His analytical approach to anatomy brought a new understanding to the study of the natural sciences. Harvey demonstrated his evidence for circulation in a Latin tract published in Germany in 1628. The only part of the system he did not describe was the invisible capillaries. He delved into the purposes of circulation and presented mathematical proof for the blood's circular route. By the time he died in 1657, Harvey had become the rare pioneer whose work was valued in his own time.

There were still greater subtleties of the vascular system too refined for Harvey's naked eye.

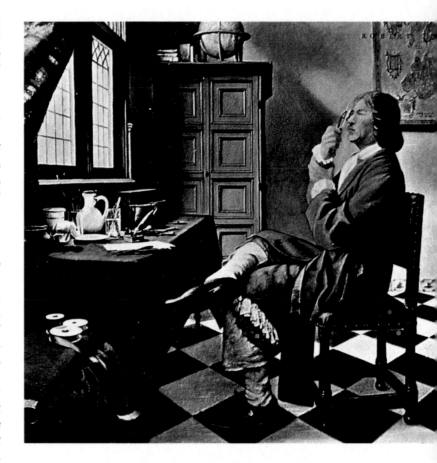

Through ingenuity and insatiable curiosity, Anton van Leeuwenhoek became one of the leading scientists of his day. A cloth merchant by profession, he ground precise lenses for his microscopes, allowing him to identify and measure red blood cells and microorganisms. Living past the age of ninety, he explored many branches of natural history, was elected to the Royal Society of London and served as a public official in the Dutch city of Delft for nearly forty years.

Anton van Leeuwenhoek

"A Person Unlearned"

Writing to the Royal Society of London in 1673, Dutch statesman Constantijn Huygens said of amateur scientist Anton van Leeuwenhoek, "He is a person unlearned in both sciences and languages." Although confident that the society would be interested in Leeuwenhoek's work, Huygens added condescendingly that Leeuwenhoek was submitting his findings for "the censure and correction of the learned."

Doubtless Huygens counted himself among the learned, and his friends over the years included philosopher René Descartes and poet John Donne. But Huygens greatly underestimated Leeuwenhoek, who in just seven years was unanimously elected to the society for his discoveries of microorganisms and red blood cells. In 1680, Huygens's own son called Leeuwenhoek "the great man of the century." By the time of his death in 1723, he was a legend of science.

A successful draper, or dry goods merchant, in the Dutch seaport of Delft, Leeuwenhoek probably became familiar with magnifying lenses by using them to inspect cloth. In time, he began to grind his own lenses and incorporated them in microscopes of his own design. Much different from the microscopes in use

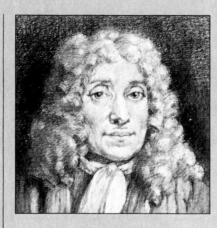

today, his consisted of lenses clamped between two flat wooden braces. He held them close to his eye and looked through the lenses toward a candle. Working alone, he focused his instruments on everything from plant lice to tooth scrapings.

After approaching the Royal Society, Leeuwenhoek flooded the scientific world with his discoveries. In 1676, he caused a sensation by announcing that he had observed creatures no larger than "the thickness of a hair in a cheese mite," thus describing man's first glimpse of microorganisms. Skeptical, the Fellows of the Royal Society compelled Leeuwenhoek to gather affidavits from several prominent citizens of Delft to verify his findings. The following year, he reported the existence of spermatozoa, modestly noting

that he hoped not to "disgust or scandalize the learned." Leeuwenhoek's discovery of parasites on fleas inspired Jonathan Swift to write:

> So naturalists observe, a flea
> Has smaller fleas that on
> him prey
> And these have smaller still
> to bite 'em;
> And so proceed *ad infinitum.*

Although other scientists had observed red blood cells, Leeuwenhoek was the first to describe them fully. In 1674, he defined them as "small red globules" and calculated that they were about "25,000 times smaller than a fine grain of sand."

In a 1683 letter, he described capillaries, which Marcello Malpighi, an Italian scientist, first saw twenty years earlier. Leeuwenhoek could not read Latin, however, so he was unaware of Malpighi's discovery. Leeuwenhoek demonstrated in 1688 that red blood cells changed shape to squeeze through small arteries.

In all, Leeuwenhoek sent 375 letters to the Royal Society, the last from his deathbed. During his lifetime he fashioned nearly 250 microscopes, but he never revealed his lens grinding secrets. As a result, his microscopes were unsurpassed for more than a hundred years.

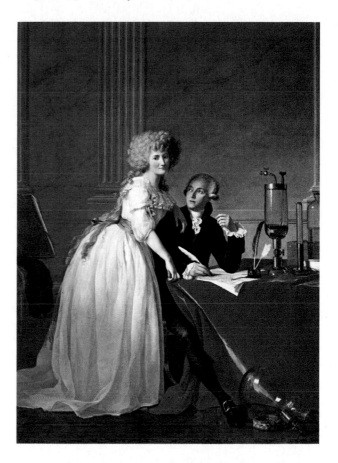

The invention of the microscope in about 1590, generally ascribed to Zacharias Janssen, a little-known Dutch lens grinder, opened up a new miniature world in the study of anatomy.

Born in 1628, the same year that Harvey published his work on the movement of the blood, Marcello Malpighi was a versatile scientist who trained his microscope on animals and plants. In 1661, he was examining the lung of a frog when he saw a network of small vessels running between the veins and the arteries. This discovery of the capillary system completed Harvey's map of the blood's circulation.

The accurate description and measurement of red corpuscles awaited Anton van Leeuwenhoek, a self-educated dry-goods merchant from Delft, Holland. Perhaps the most ingenious amateur scientist the world has ever known, he studied the red blood cells of mammals, birds and fish and determined that these were the cells that produced the red color of blood. Leeuwenhoek examined his own blood every day to gauge his health. If his blood appeared darker and thicker than normal, he drank four cups of coffee for breakfast instead of two and six cups of tea in the afternoon instead of his usual three.

As scientific inquiry grew more sophisticated, the manifold functions of the blood were revealed. The seventeenth-century invention of the air pump, which drew air out of glass chambers to create a vacuum, proved that some substance in air sustained life. British scientist Robert Boyle found in 1661 that a candle and a mouse expired simultaneously when air was withdrawn from a glass vacuum chamber. It was not until the 1770s, though, that another Briton, Joseph Priestley, isolated oxygen as the component in air that brightened dark venous blood. He did not fully realize the importance of his discovery, but the French scientist Antoine Lavoisier did.

Using advanced techniques of chemistry, he showed that the body, like fire, consumed nutrients and gave off heat. It was Lavoisier who gave oxygen its name. His career was cut short, however. In 1792, in the early years of the French Revolution, a colleague recommended that the Academy of Sciences be purged of reactionaries. Lavoisier, appointed to an administrative position under royal rule, was arrested and tried as an enemy of France for "mixing tobacco with water and ingredients harmful to the health of its citizens." An official of the revolutionary tribunal that tried him remarked, "The Republic has no need for the learned." The revolution was based on the strength of rationalism, but with the execution of Lavoisier, it extinguished its brightest light of reason. On May 8, 1794, the same day as his trial, he was guillotined.

Pascal, the philosopher and mathematician, once said, "Rivers are highways that move on, and bear us whither we wish to go." Channeled within the banks of veins and arteries, continually replenished to maintain a smooth current, the blood stream can be said to resemble a river. Through the ages of man, blood's magical red fluid has often seemed more spirit than matter. The life-giving breath, we now know, is oxygen, only one of many substances carried in the blood.

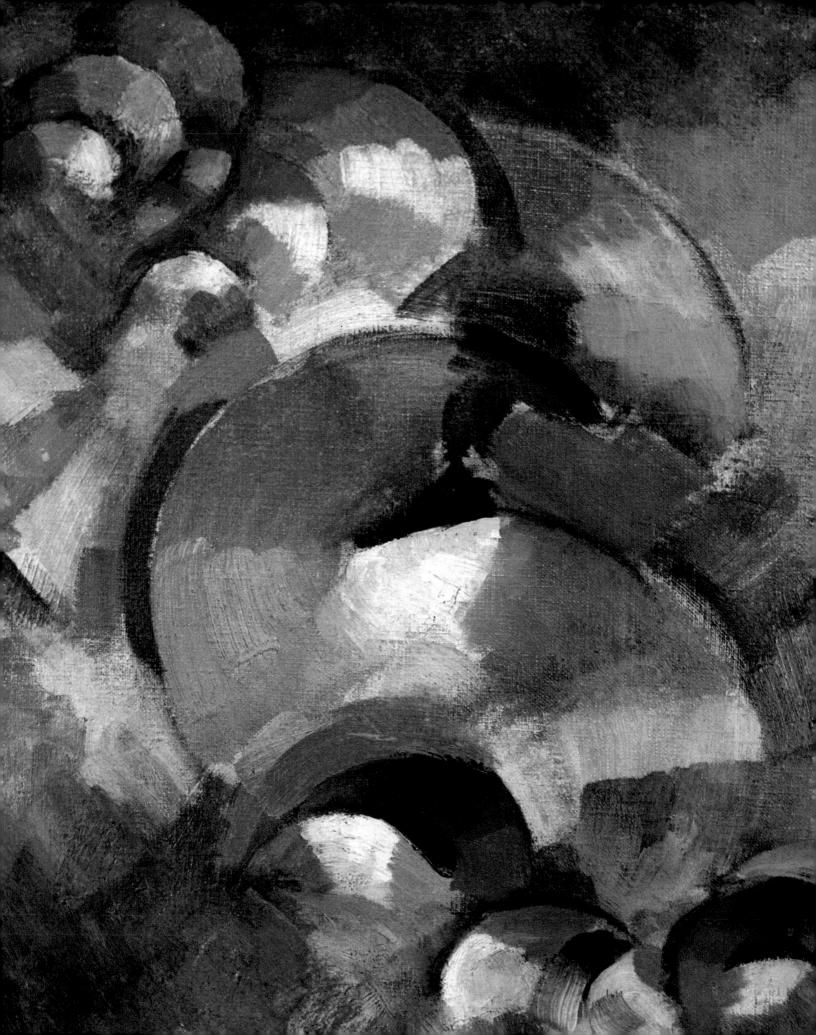

Chapter 2

The Liquid Tissue

All blood is alike ancient," an old English proverb says. Modern scientific theories suggest that all blood may indeed have common ancestry in primal seas of the Cambrian era. During this time, some half a billion years ago, the first life forms are believed to have emerged from the sea to take up residence on land. Then only a third as salty as they are today, the waters contained the same proportion of minerals and salts contained in human blood. Primordial oceans were blood's prototype but, by necessity, blood grew thicker than water.

For all its similarities in origin, composition and duty, blood is as unique from person to person as are hair, skin and bone. It carries a stamp of genetic blueprints like all our physical features. As these differences have come to be better understood, the life-giving fluid has become the most easily and widely shared of human tissues. It saves lives daily.

While blood is not the most watery of our tissues, it is the only liquid one. Blood does for man what the mighty oceans do for the smallest forms of life. To perform its vital functions, it must move swiftly and powerfully. A little more than half actual fluid, blood is crowded with a society of diverse, solid cells, each assigned specific duties and coexisting in critical proportion. Should the population of only one element fall, life would be threatened.

The River's Abundance

The roster of blood's daily chores is staggering. It supplies the vital gas, oxygen, to each of the other sixty trillion cells in the body. It transports food, wastes and hormonal messengers. It rushes to the stomach after meals, the lungs during exertion and the face in embarrassment. It cools when and where there is overheating and warms where there is danger of freezing. And it defends the body, destroying alien invaders. If the wall of

Surging whirls of color in Morgan Russell's Cosmic Synchromy, *painted in 1914, evoke the intense vitality of life's current, blood. A host of myriad performers in rhythmic harmony, blood unites solid elements in a river of purposeful tissue.*

Blood will settle into three distinct, proportional layers when treated with salt. The transparent yellow layer at top is plasma, the liquid portion of blood. Through it travel solid elements, here enlarged for illustration. White blood cells settle in the narrow white band in the center, and red blood cells, which give blood its crimson color, fall to the bottom of the flask. Red cells outnumber white 600 to one.

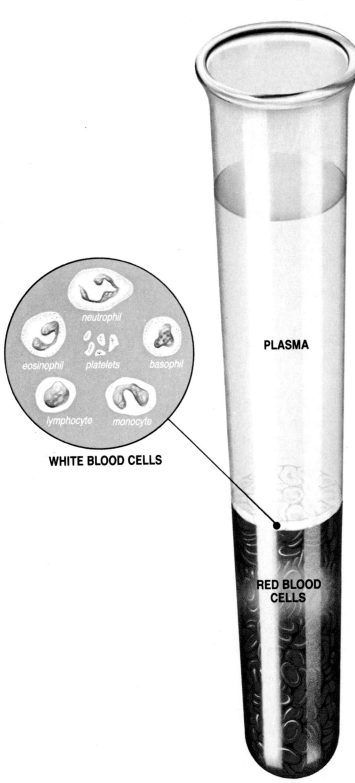

WHITE BLOOD CELLS

neutrophil

eosinophil

platelets

basophil

lymphocyte

monocyte

PLASMA

RED BLOOD
CELLS

a blood vessel bursts, blood itself quickly seals and mends the vessel so that massive bacterial invasion does not take place. In short, blood is the river enriching the continent called man.

Scientists are still looking for ways to "dissect" the liquid tissue. Long ago, in the fourth century B.C., Hippocrates observed that blood will settle into three distinct layers when treated with salt and left undisturbed in a transparent flask for several hours. The largest layer, at the top, is a clear, straw-colored liquid. The middle layer forms a narrow band of white. The heaviest, settled on the bottom, is red.

Stilling the Current

Today, scientists call the clear portion of blood plasma. About 92 percent water, plasma is the blood's solvent. Salts, minerals, sugars, fats and proteins — all the foodstuffs of life — find passage through plasma. There, too, bicarbonates wait to meet and escort poisonous wastes to the kidneys, the body's efficient filters.

The most important ingredients in plasma are three proteins — albumin, globulins and fibrinogen. Using meat and milk for raw materials, the liver manufactures all of them, not to be used as food for the body, but to serve a variety of other functions. Albumin, the most plentiful, is similar to egg white and gives blood its gummy texture. The presence of these large proteins keeps the water concentration of blood low, so that water diffuses readily from tissues into the blood. The globulins — alpha, beta and gamma — number half the albumin proteins. Globulins transport certain other proteins. Gamma globulins, the antibodies of the blood, give man immunity to disease. Fibrinogen, a mere 3 percent of plasma's proteins, is an indispensable link in the chain of reactions that leads to blood's clotting. It forms a web of fine protein fibers that bind blood cells together, creating a bridge over which injured tissue can rebuild itself while the blood stream flows, uninterrupted, beneath it.

The workings of the plasma proteins are still quite mysterious to scientists. Aside from routine duties, they can alter their functions readily, like versatile handymen in the maintenance of the blood. Should the blood's acidity waver, disrupting the normal rate of chemical reactions in the body's cells, the proteins can act either as acid or base to correct it. They "lubricate" the blood so that it flows smoothly. And they can transport other passengers — from fat-soluble vitamins to hormones and carbohydrates. Should the body run short of food, plasma proteins offer themselves up for digestion to sustain the body temporarily. Physiologist Leo Vroman likened the search for all the roles of plasma proteins to "a dense jungle" where "the blind hunters in it cannot hope to catch any rare and rarely singing bird alive. We can shoot at its voice and hear it stop or change into shrieks of fright. Many a protein changes its song after it has been caught, and turns out to be a mockingbird."

There are also minerals in plasma — the salts, metals and inorganic compounds that measure in uncannily similar proportions to the same elements thought by scientists to have existed in the ancient Cambrian seas. The first one-celled residents of those seas had circulatory systems as vast as the ocean itself with its almost limitless supplies. Abundant in oceans, oxygen diffused effortlessly into these single-celled creatures, and allowed them to carry out the combustion of foods to make energy, the metabolic process we call life. Just as easily, the sea absorbed carbon dioxide, waste product of metabolism.

The same process still serves simple sea creatures. In more complex life, individual cells are building blocks, some of which are cut off from direct contact with water. Circulatory systems, scientists think, evolved hand in hand with structural complexities. The sponge has an open circulatory system, a network of pores and tunnels that allows each cell intimate contact with the oxygen-rich sea water.

Pliers of Cargo

Even though oxygen can dissolve in plasma, just as it does in sea water, and even though the plasma circulates everywhere in the body, it can only carry about 1 percent of all the oxygen that our bodies demand. Red blood cells provide the other 99 percent. Called erythrocytes, the red blood cells form the bottom layer of settled blood that Hippocrates observed so long ago. Although they constitute about 45 percent of the blood, red cells are the most abundant cells in the body. Their single task is to shuttle oxygen to tissue and remove carbon dioxide. Rounded disks with nearly hollowed-out centers, red blood cells are sturdy but highly flexible sacs that can squeeze through the narrowest passages in the blood stream without rupturing. They are made mainly of water and the red protein called hemoglobin, which is so highly concentrated in individual red cells that it almost forms crystals.

Marrow, the Master Shipwright

The production of the cargo shuttlers is a mobile process assigned to specific sites throughout life. In the womb during the first weeks of gestation, red cells are made in the yolk sac of the embryo. By four-and-a-half months after conception, the liver, spleen and lymph nodes have taken over production. Late in pregnancy, the task of manufacturing has been transferred to the marrow of bones, where it will continue for the rest of life. It is an example of what British physiologist E. H. Starling called "the wisdom of the body" to house this vital process in such armored quarters. In adults, the marrow of the skull, ribs and spine manufactures most red blood cells, but any bone marrow in the body can be called upon to contribute in an emergency.

When tissue runs short of oxygen, a messenger hormone called erythropoietin travels to the marrow. There, the messenger signals a primitive cell — so named because it has yet to develop fully — to begin growth. Jolted from dormancy, the cell becomes a rubriblast that splits in two. Each of the pair in turn divides until there are sixteen red blood cells. Inside every cell, the making of hemoglobin is already under way. It continues until the concentration of the protein becomes 95 percent of the dry weight of the cell. As this saturation point approaches, the cell expels its nucleus, the control center for metabolism, growth and reproduction. It is an act of self-sterilization; the red blood cell will never reproduce again. Indeed, without a nucleus, the cell is often called a corpuscle. As if visibly bearing the signature of this act, the cell now looks like a pinched disk. The new, characteristic shape

31

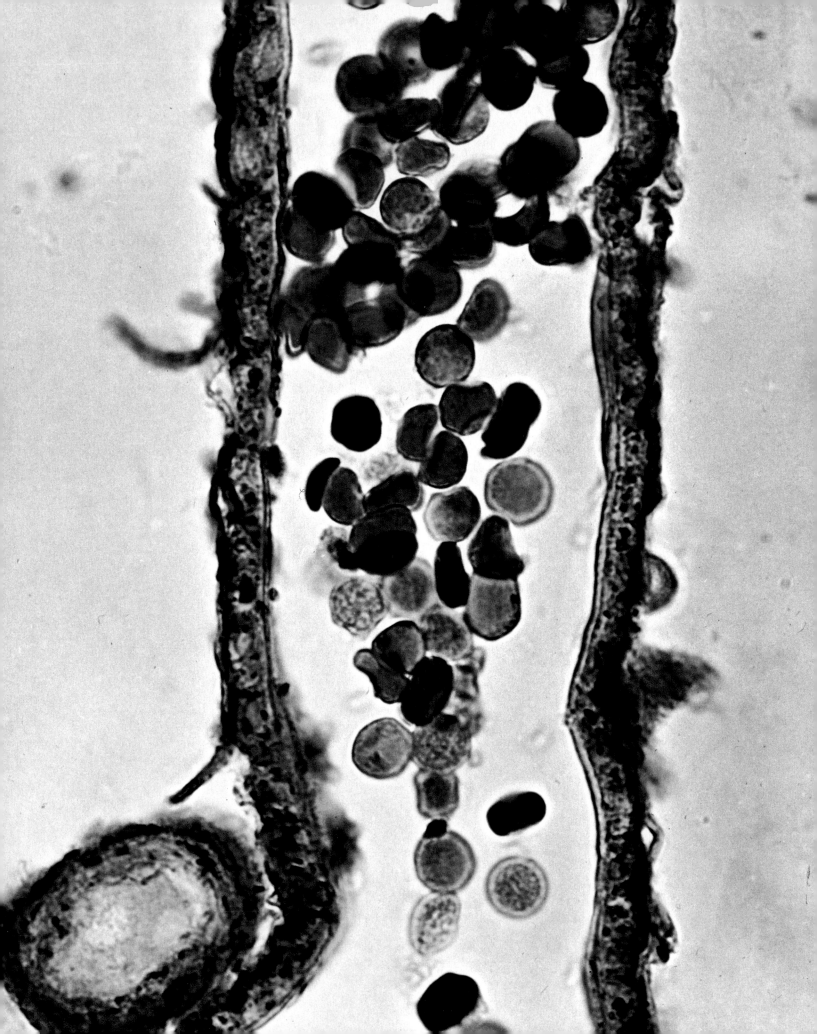

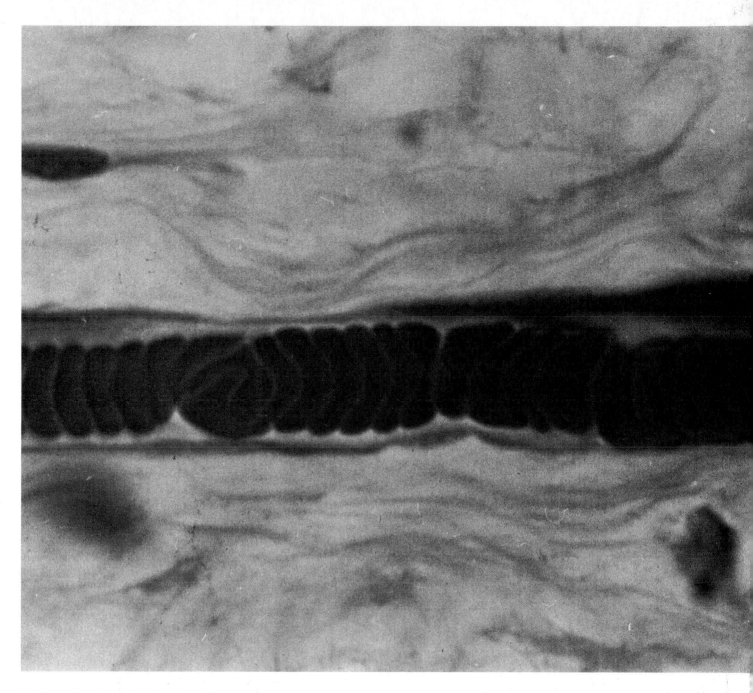

Fueling all motion in the body, red blood cells carrying oxygen, left, cascade through a single capillary to reach the cerebellum, the brain's control center for motor coordination and balance. Above, when forced through narrower straits feeding tooth pulp, the oxygen carriers stack up against each other like coins to maintain the steady flow of blood. This phenomenon, the Rouleaux formation, can occur spontaneously anywhere in the blood stream.

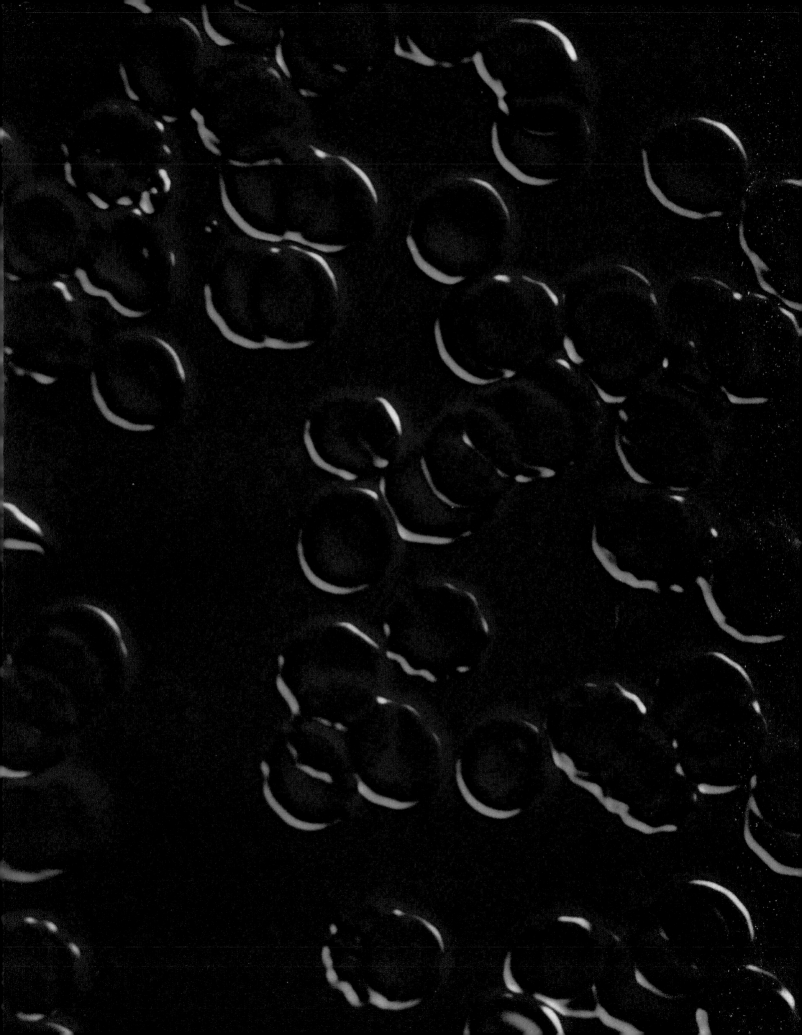

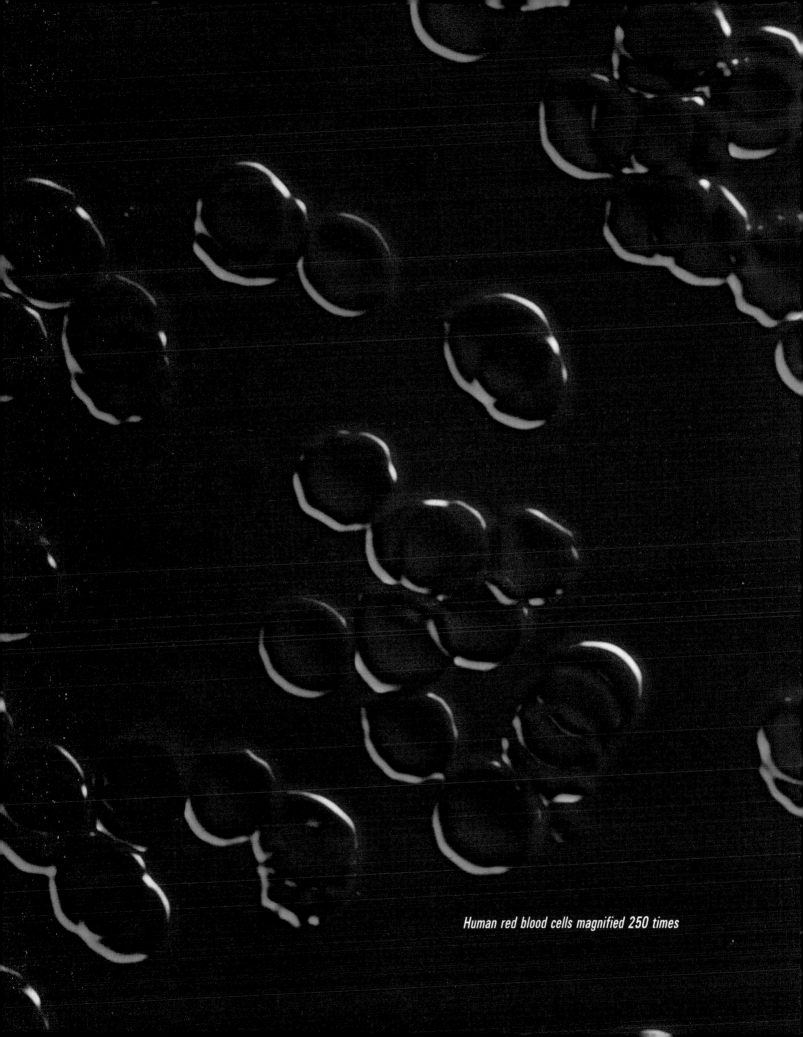

Human red blood cells magnified 250 times

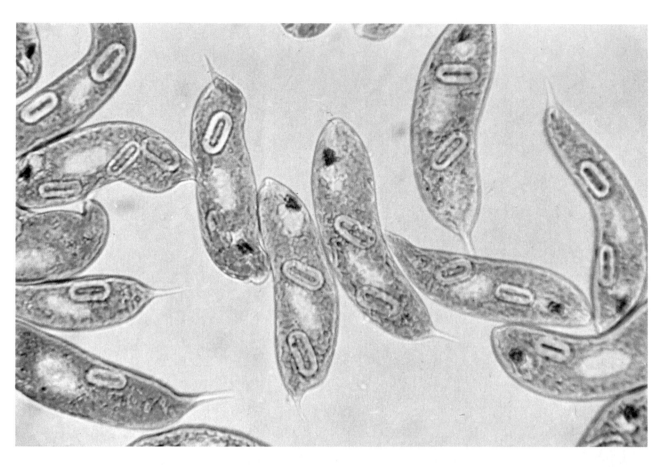

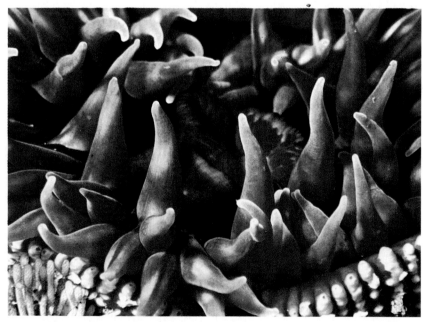

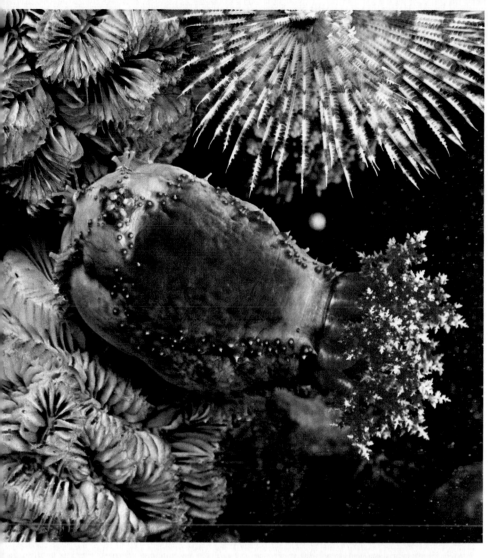

These seemingly simple creatures of the sea gather their nutrients from the waters they live in. Boasting circulatory systems infinitely more vast than man's, they are, nevertheless, bound to an aquatic life. The single-celled euglena, above left, can synthesize food from sunlight like a plant, or hunt and eat smaller creatures like an animal. A hollow tube runs through the length of the sea cucumber, above right, providing this cousin of the starfish with a hydraulic vascular system that not only nourishes but also gives it a means of propulsion. Sea anemones, bottom left and right, produce a chemical repellent that wards off predators and eventually hardens to form coral reefs. Inexorably dependent upon the sea, these are among the billions of her residents who have no need for blood.

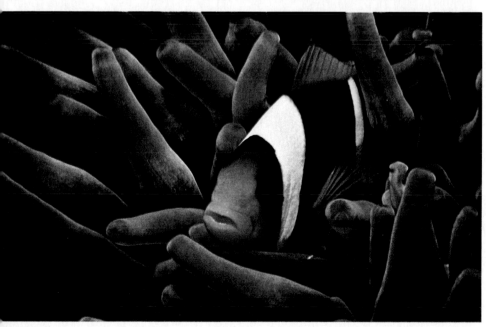

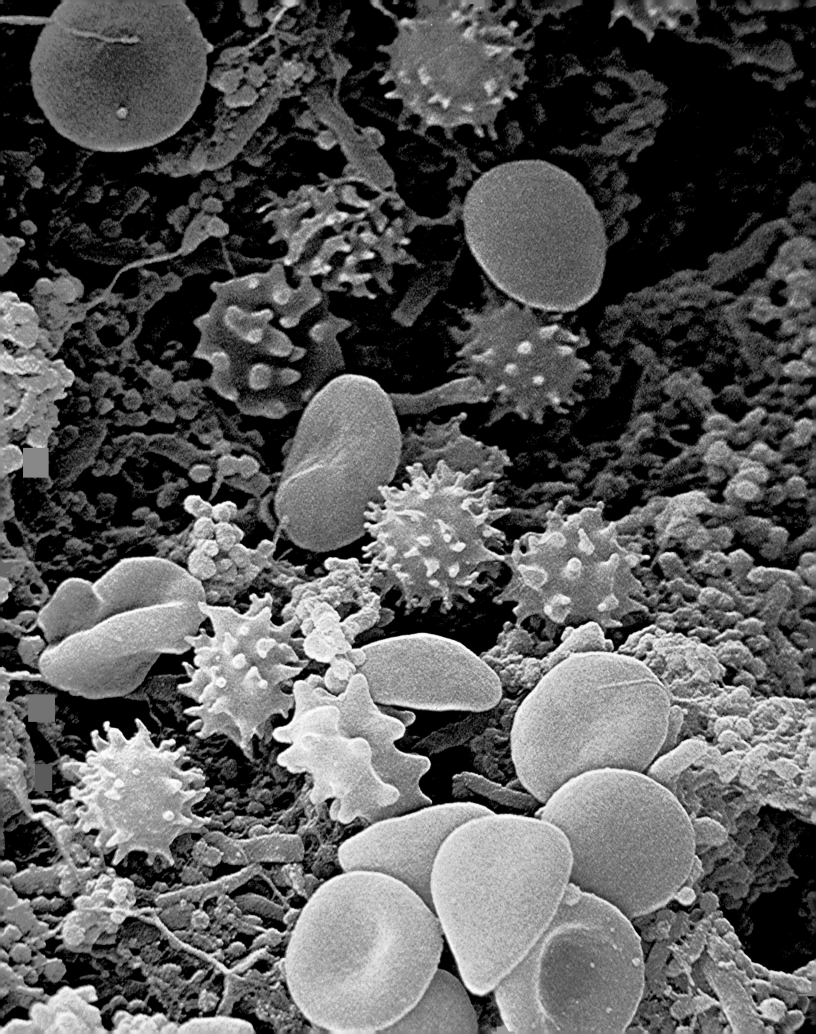

Red blood cells, left, react to high acidity by swelling into spiked balls called echinocytes, from the Greek meaning "sea urchin." Bone marrow, below, is the blood cells' place of birth, nursery and graveyard.

Below, in the birth sequence of a red blood cell, a process that takes six days to complete, the forming cell convulses, belching out its nucleus on day three, top. It continues to writhe into its final disk shape.

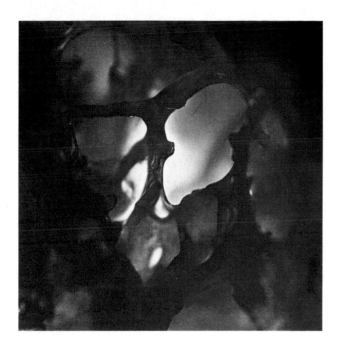

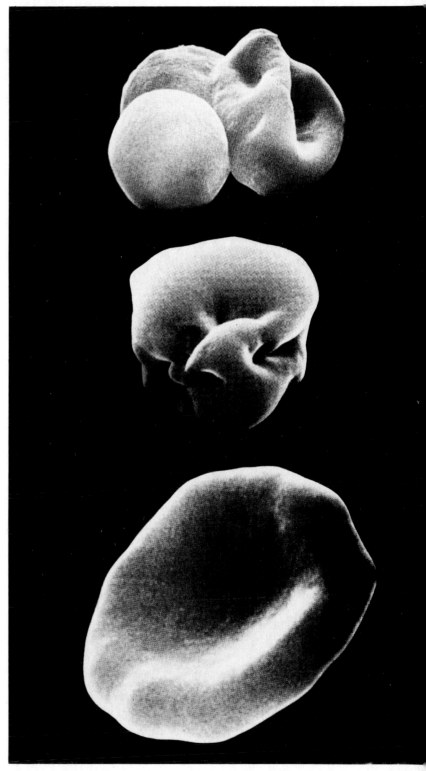

greatly increases the cell's surface area and, thus, its oxygen-carrying potential. The production of a corpuscle takes 6 days to complete. Yet the cell will live for only 120 days. In a typical lifetime, bone marrow will manufacture more than half a ton of red blood cells in this manner.

Why not produce the hemoglobin carrier and let it make its own way through the plasma? The answer, scientists have discovered, lies in nature's design. Without the protection of the cell, hemoglobin flowing in the blood stream would be filtered out quickly. Each red blood cell contains roughly 270 million hemoglobin molecules. The protein itself is complex in structure, for it must bind well with oxygen, but not too well. It must load oxygen at the surface of the lungs, hold on to the precious cargo during passage through the blood's swift rapids and cramped tributaries but, at just the right moment, unload the oxygen wherever the body's cells need it.

The hemoglobin molecule looks like an elaborate piece of jewelry constructed of four entwined chains of amino acids, the stuff of proteins. In the middle of each chain lies the heme, a ring of carbon, hydrogen and nitrogen atoms. Heme provides a setting for the centerpiece — a single atom of iron. It is the iron atom

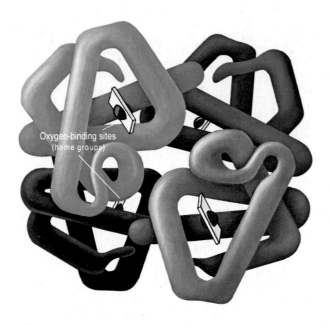

Oxygen-binding sites
(heme groups)

Elaborate mechanism of oxygen transport for the body, the four-chained hemoglobin molecule, above, is made from more than 10,000 atoms. Yet, when fully laden, the molecule will carry but four pairs of oxygen atoms. One of the body's largest proteins, hemoglobin is built around four atoms of iron, which act like oxygen magnets. The molecule binds the gas firmly enough for its trip from the lungs to body tissue but loosely enough to release it at just the right moment. Each red blood cell holds 300 million of these vital protein molecules.

that binds to oxygen. With four such studs, a hemoglobin molecule can therefore carry four oxygen molecules. But this in itself does not explain the complex structure of the molecule. If iron were all that were needed to carry oxygen, then the chains and settings would be unnecessary. The framework's configuration effectively separates the iron and oxygen. If they floated freely in the blood stream, they would bind together irreversibly. Sheltered in the network of the heme, the iron atom is somewhat "occupied" in all the interrelationships with the atoms surrounding it. The influence exerted by its nearest neighbors, especially a certain nitrogen atom, dilutes iron's attraction to oxygen, assuring that the relationship is only a temporary one. The craftsmanship of the hemoglobin molecule allows red blood cells to pick up oxygen where it is most plentiful — in the lungs — and release it where it is scarcest in the body's other tissues.

Pirates Along the Stream

The structure of the hemoglobin molecule, however, is not foolproof. It is ideal for discriminating among the gases found naturally in our atmosphere, and prefers oxygen to the more plentiful nitrogen. Yet it has not "learned" to deal with impurities, such as carbon monoxide, a pervasive, toxic by-product of the gasoline engine. The iron of the heme, more confused than fickle, prefers carbon monoxide to oxygen. Its bond with carbon monoxide is 230 times stronger than its bond with oxygen. Not only does iron prefer carbon monoxide but it makes a bond so tight that none of the body's chemistry can break it up. The poison accumulates, hijacking the red cells that continue making their rounds but do nothing for the body's oxygen-starved tissue. If the air in an enclosed room were to contain only half of 1 percent carbon monoxide, a person inside would die in less than a half-hour. While his body's tissues might send out dire messages to his bone marrow to produce more red cells, the six-day process would be futile. New cells would only be fooled in the same way.

Blood that has been occupied with carbon monoxide is a bright, cherry red color, a much brighter red than normally oxygenated blood.

Ominous by-product of technology,
air pollution paints a grim horizon.
Traces of manmade contaminating
wastes scatter to the most remote
corners of wilderness, and find their
way into man's own blood stream.

When blood has delivered oxygen to tissues, it loads up carbon dioxide and turns blue. Blood's chameleonlike properties helped save a president's life. In March 1981, when Ronald Reagan was shot in Washington, D.C., his bodyguard pushed him into the back seat of the presidential limousine. The president insisted he was all right. But the agent later reported, "There was blood coming from his mouth and it was bright red. . . . I knew it was coming from his lungs." He told the driver to head for the hospital.

Man's oxygen transport system is remarkably adaptable and responsive. At higher altitudes, as the air gets thinner, blood cells show up at the lungs as usual but find less oxygen and return to the tissues only partially laden. The tissues complain via hormones to the bone marrow, which immediately begins to manufacture more red blood cells. The red cell concentration of a person traveling from sea-level Los Angeles to mile-high Denver will soon increase 10 percent. Mountain sickness starts at about 10,000 feet; above this altitude, careful acclimatization is necessary to avoid mountain sickness. At 18,500 feet, air pressure is reduced to half that of sea level, and the number of red blood cells will, given time, increase by 50 percent.

The red blood cell is a tireless and faithful servant. Undisturbed by disease or infection, it will wear itself out with work — making 75,000 trips between the lungs and the body's tissues — in four months. Ragged and exhausted, sensing its hour of death, the red cell seeks its place of birth to die. In the bone marrow is the agent of its demise. Relative turned cannibal, a large white blood cell enshrouds and ingests the weary red one, breaking it down to raw materials once again. The white cell spews out what remains of the destroyed cell for the manufacture of more red ones. Thus, the red blood cell ends its service in rebirth. Chief among its raw materials is the precious iron, which the body hoards. Three hundred billion red blood cells, about 1 percent of the body's total number, are so lost and replaced each day — the equivalent of changing the world's population every twenty minutes.

Not all red blood cells are so neatly disposed of. The blood stream carries many dead blood

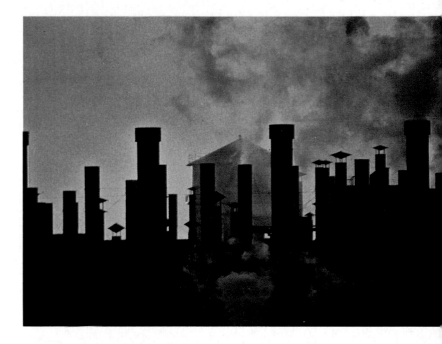

cells — ruptured, emptied sacs — that it sometimes deposits elsewhere in the body. These ghost cells drift and can wend their way into the eyes. Their littered remains are the white spots in our sight called "floaters" that circulate in the clear fluid of the eye's sphere.

The River Patrol

The large white scavengers waiting for the red cells in the marrow are more than grim reapers. They are members of a vast army of blood cells, the leukocytes. Outnumbered by the red cells — 600 to 1 — they form the narrow white layer Hippocrates had seen. With five divisions, leukocytes are the standing troops that defend the blood stream, and thus the whole body, from deadly microscopic invaders.

Three of the five white cells have a granular appearance. These are the neutrophils, eosinophils and basophils. The other two, the lymphocytes and monocytes, have smooth, nongranular bodies. More than half of the white army stands guard throughout the body; the rest patrol, coursing along the stream. All have mobility. All can creep along the walls of the blood stream to stalk their prey, independent of the moving current. They defend the body against the bacteria

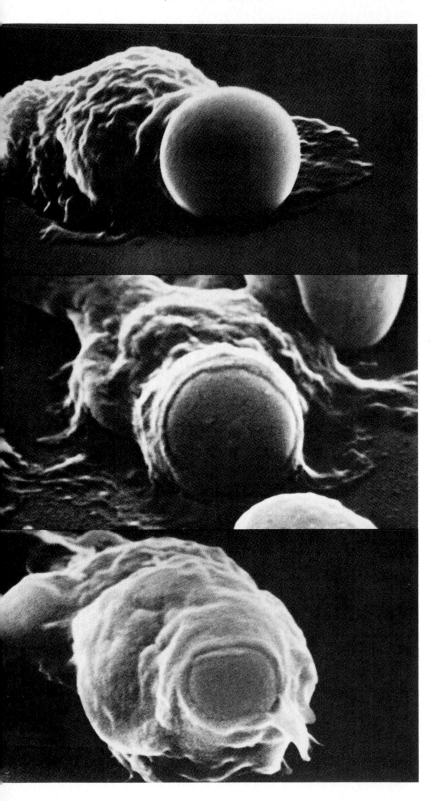

of everyday life, the viruses, fungi and parasites that can accumulate in the body's openings and infiltrate the blood stream. Such ordinary impurities, unchecked, would cause severe illness. Others, more virulent and aggressive foes, can break through the front-line guards to wreak havoc in the blood. Normally, the white blood cells respond like a rapid-deployment force. Their lives are hard, dangerous and short.

The leukocyte army is a team of specialists. Depending on the nature of the invader, they perform two basic tasks. Basophils and some lymphocytes act like mines. In the presence of an alien, they erupt and spew out chemicals that trigger inflammation: the vessels swell, other proteins seal off the area, trapping the enemy, and the walls of the vessels grow sticky. Their rupturing inflames the area and sets the stage for the battle. The neutrophils, eosinophils or monocytes then arrive to engulf the trapped alien. This process is called phagocytosis, derived from the Greek word meaning "to eat." Some phagocytes just swallow up the enemy to neutralize it; others take their work a step further by breaking it down and digesting it. All are ravenous. A typical phagocyte will continue to consume toxic bacteria, debris or other foreign matter until, in effect, it dies from overeating.

A phagocyte obeys three basic signals that keep it from eating everything it encounters in the blood stream. First, since most of the regular passengers through the blood stream have smooth surfaces, a particle with a rough texture will automatically be engulfed. The second signal is an electrical one. Most resident substances in the body have negative surface charges, while aliens, in general, have positively charged ones. The attraction between white cell and invader occurs almost instantly. The third signal is chemical, one that tags the invader with antibodies — proteins manufactured by the white cells. The antibodies mark the invader a victim of that potent defense system called immunity.

The bone marrow and lymph glands continually produce and maintain a reserve of white blood cells. A leukocyte that patrols the blood for a few hours — a normal, active lifetime — can wait outside of the stream for more than six days before it gets its cue to enter. The reserve is vital. There are not many white cells in the healthy blood stream, and those that are there are well occupied with routine chores. When a parasite or virus invades and begins to colonize, reserves are unleashed and the manufacturing of vast quantities of the appropriate white cells feverishly begins. It is this heated production that causes fever. Aching bones and sore throat (from the swelling of the lymph glands) are signs that the body is busy fighting back.

Because white cells are very specific for various illnesses, counting their numbers helps doctors diagnose patients. If the percentage of monocytes — normally 5 — rises to 20 or 30, the illness could be Rocky Mountain spotted fever, typhus or tuberculosis. Neutrophils, the most numerous white cells, normally constitute about 60 percent; a rise above 75 might indicate pneumonia or appendicitis. And when parasites — such as Trichinella, found in raw pork — invade the blood, the count of eosinophils can rise from less than 3 percent to more than 50.

Also part of the blood's defense system are small cells known as platelets. When a blood vessel is cut, platelets rush to the site. They swell into odd, irregular shapes, grow sticky, clog at the cut and create a plug. If the cut is too large for platelets to stop escaping blood, they send out signals that initiate clotting. Our smallest vessels rupture hundreds of times each day, but platelets alone are able to make the necessary repairs.

Pumping the Tributaries

Long before mankind had any knowledge of the myriad specialists at work in the blood, he was convinced that it was the source of life. "The life of the flesh is in the blood," proclaims the Book of Leviticus. Man has persisted in trying to turn the mysteries of blood to his advantage. If blood was the source of life, then it was also the source of health and illness. By letting bad blood flow out, illness would dissipate; by replacing it with fresh blood, health could be restored. In tribute to this superstition, blood flowed for centuries in the name of the sacred and the profane. It was not until the twentieth century that man made the process of transfusion safe.

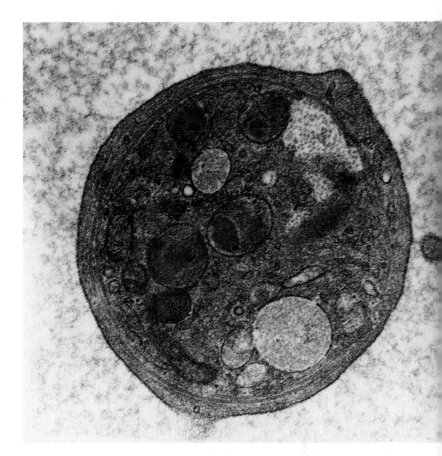

The blood stream's smallest and most versatile cell, a platelet — magnified 45,000 times — rushes to seal broken vessels anywhere in the body. If the vessel is large, the platelets simultaneously send out chemical signals that initiate the complex clotting process. Every day platelets alone suffice in the repair of millions of ruptured capillaries, making clotting unnecessary.

Medea, mythological witch, tests
her youth potion with a barren olive
twig, which promptly sprouts spring
growth. Such legends sprang from
beliefs that blood mediated youth
and age, sickness and health.

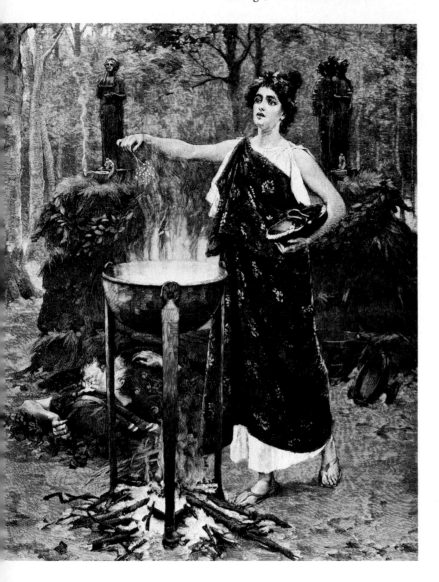

In 43 B.C., the poet Ovid told the tale of a re-sourceful witch, Medea. As a favor to woo her mortal lover, Jason, she rejuvenated his aging father. She cut his throat, drained out his blood and replaced it with a magic potion made of

> Roots, seeds, and flowers, and saps dark-hued
>   were there,
> And blossoms that Thessalian lowlands bare;
> Gems, by the farthest lands of dawn supplied,
> And sands, well washed by ocean's ebbing
>   tide;
> Frosts, which beneath the nightlong moon
>   were sought,
> And flesh of owls, and wings accurst, she
>   brought;
> And entrails of the wizzard wolf, who can
> Whene'er he will, assume the shape of man;
> Liver of long-lived stag; and, wafer-thin,
> The Libyan river serpent's scaly skin;
> A raven's head, surviving centuries nine —
> All these ingredients did the witch combine.

In Rome, gladiators drank the blood of their fallen opponents so that courage would not flow into the sand to be wasted. At the end of the games, spectators joined in the partaking. And Jesus of Nazareth bound his disciples to an ever-lasting covenant by entreating them to drink wine that represented his blood.

Bloodletting, the draining of blood to purge the body of illness, was a popular remedy as long ago as the twelfth century. A manuscript of the time credited the practice with healing diverse ailments. Bloodletting, it stated, "makes the mind sincere, aids the memory, reforms the bladder, warms the marrows, opens the hearing, removes nausea, invites digestion, evokes the voice, moves the bowels and removes anxiety." For lack of knowledge bloodletting persisted. In the same year that Columbus discovered America, Pope Innocent VIII lay dying. When all known medical remedies failed, his physicians took blood from three boys, and gave it to the pope to drink. The boys died and, shortly after, so did the pope.

In the seventeenth century, science bested superstition. Englishman William Harvey proved that blood moved in a closed system and that it circulated from the pumping action of the heart. The Royal Society of London celebrated his suc-

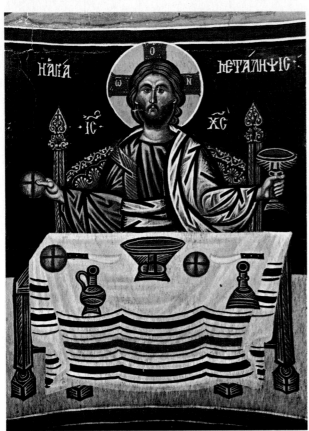

Enriching the ancient belief that blood contained the potent power of life, Jesus of Nazareth, left, holds a chalice of wine representing his blood — a new covenant by which man could conquer sin and death.

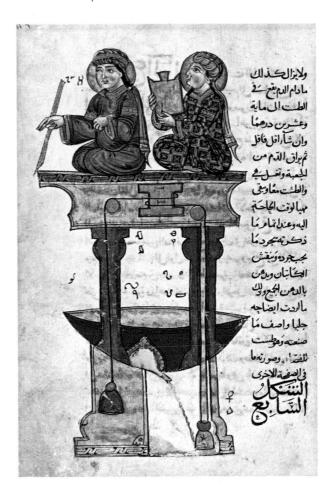

cess, championed his theory and immediately set out to elaborate on it. Architect and anatomist Christopher Wren demonstrated Harvey's theory. To perform the experiment, he made a syringe, one of the first, from silver tubes and an animal's bladder. Injecting "divers substances" directly into the veins of dogs, Wren watched as "the animals were immediately purged, vomited, intoxicated, killed or revived, according to the quality of the liquor injected." So recorded the Royal Society's secretary. The learned gentlemen concluded from these experiments that blood carried medicines to all parts of the body.

Elsewhere in England, a more profound experiment was under way. Oxford physician Richard Lower joined the artery of a healthy dog to the vein of another that had been bled almost to death. The failing dog immediately regained its vigor. Lower later claimed such transfusion would best serve to replace blood that had been lost from injury or hemorrhage. But the medical world seized upon it as a treatment for the mentally disturbed, in hopes of purging the foul and destructive humors that plagued the insane. In the fall of 1667, the Royal Society invited Lower to attempt his experiment on a human being. Somewhat reluctantly, he agreed.

An ancient art if not a science, bloodletting was a popular form of healing ills. Counting each precious drop, two Arab scribes sit on top of a fourteenth-century bloodletting device. The script says they must alternately count three gram units of blood — called dirhams — until twenty ounces have been drained from a patient's blood, contained in the basin below. The system of pulleys is attached to the scribes' arms and moves their pens as the brass basin fills.

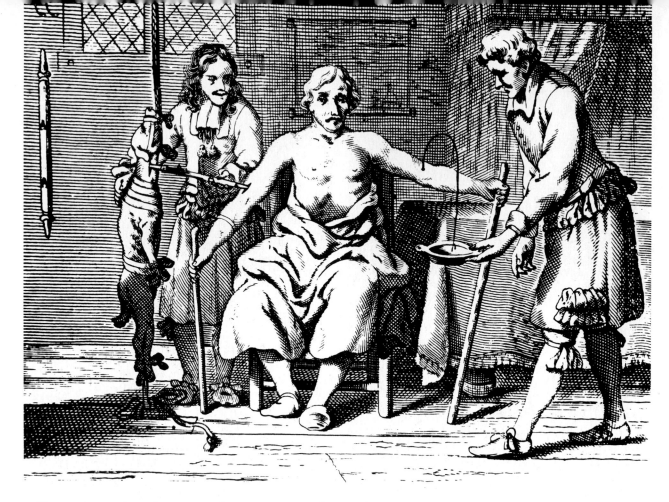

The society selected a young clergyman named Arthur Coga, a man "whose brain was considered a little too warm," and who was "willing to suffer the experiment of transfusion to be tryed on himself for a guiny." Lower drained seven ounces of Coga's "unbalanced" blood from the surface vein inside the elbow. In the vein, he then inserted a silver tube connected to the artery of a sheep. Coga and animal remained connected for two minutes. Six days later, the patient appeared before the society and reported that he felt much better. His Latin was intact, a sure sign to the society's members that the young man had regained his wits. Coga received a second transfusion a few weeks later with equal success. The only discomfort he experienced was a hangover from a drinking bout after the operation.

The society's secretary left no report as to whether or not the man's overheated brain ever cooled. But the demonstration quickly became the hottest topic of conversation in European society. It was even mentioned in Samuel Pepys's *Diary*. Across the English Channel, in the summer of that same year, Jean-Baptiste Denis had cured a fifteen-year-old boy of a recurring fever by transfusing him with nine ounces of lamb's blood. Outraged over the English claim for the milestone, the French medical world declared France first in the experiment. But less than a month after the controversy started, Denis fell into a scandal that was to put a damper on all transfusions for the next century and a half.

Believing the procedure would invigorate him, a Scandinavian nobleman sought Denis's treatment. But the northerner died from the transfusion. Later, Denis used the blood of a "gentle calf" to "dampen" another man's maniacal spirits. The patient calmed down, and a few days later Denis repeated the treatment. But this time, the man complained of pain in his kidneys and arm, tightness in his chest, sweating, and urine that was "black as soot." Doctors now recognize this documented report as a typical transfusion reaction: the antibodies manufactured from the first transfusion were sufficiently developed to attack the second invasion of foreign blood. The man recovered, but within a short time his wife dragged him back to Denis. She insisted Denis once again calm her husband's foul temper, but her husband would not cooperate. The next night the man died and his wife charged Denis with the murder. In court, the defense proved that the woman had poisoned her husband with arsenic. Denis was exonerated, but transfusion was not.

Within the next decade London, Paris and Rome banned transfusions. Even though forbidden, it was still practiced. But its results would remain unpredictable until other scientific discoveries could improve the technique. In 1777, Frenchman Antoine Lavoisier, father of modern chemistry, demonstrated that the purpose of breathing was to gather oxygen from air. Iron had already been found in the blood, but it was not until the 1850s that German physiologist and chemist Otto Funke discovered hemoglobin. Twelve years later, his compatriot Ernst Felix Hoppe-Seyler gave hemoglobin its name and demonstrated its ability to take up and discharge oxygen. In the early 1900s, British obstetrician James Blundell performed transfusions on women hemorrhaging from childbirth. From his successes, he concluded that for human transfusions "only human blood should be employed."

A natural function of blood — clotting — still remained an obstacle to safe transfusion. When removed from a donor or sent through pipes, red blood began to gel within minutes. Scientists tried various means to overcome its clotting. Whipping blood with an egg whisk and then removing the clot that had formed was a method made popular in France. Another technique was the joining a donor's artery to a recipient's vein.

This delicate surgery took place on a kitchen table in New York City in 1908. Alexis Carrel, a French surgeon studying animal-organ transplants at The Rockefeller Institute, sewed a father's artery to the vein of his newborn daughter. The infant, who had been hemorrhaging badly, promptly recovered. At the time, a bill banning vivisection for experiments on living animals was about to go before the New York State Senate. But when the New York newspapers heralded Carrel's successful transfusion as the result of a skill perfected on laboratory animals, the bill was resoundingly squashed.

Still, there was a mysterious obstacle to safe transfusions. Standard techniques too often produced adverse reactions. And no one knew why. The answer was provided by a young Viennese researcher at the beginning of the century.

Karl Landsteiner set out to prove that there were individual differences in human blood. He

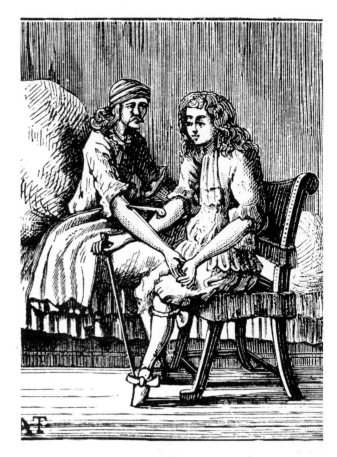

Two seventeenth-century prints depict early attempts to share blood as a primitive means of restoring health. Opposite, a dog unwillingly demonstrated that man's best friend was not necessarily his best donor. Above, the more sensible transfusion between human beings, still evoked equally unpredictable and violent reactions. Transfusion would remain unsafe for the next 300 years.

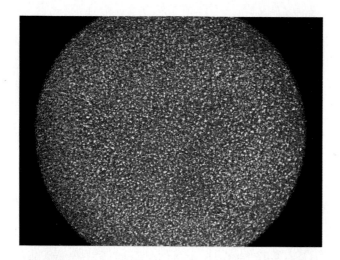

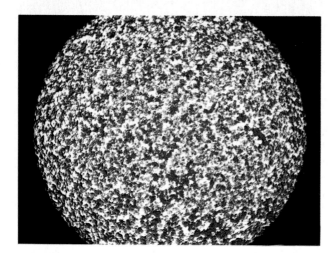

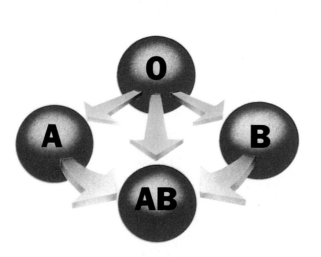

used a simple, direct method. Landsteiner took blood samples from himself and five laboratory assistants. Separating each sample into its plasma and red blood cell components, he then mixed the individual plasmas with the different samples of red cells. Landsteiner noted two reactions. The red cells, introduced to foreign plasma, either clumped together or they did not. He charted the results and repeated the experiment with more volunteers, eventually identifying three types of human blood. Two of Landsteiner's assistants, Alfred von Decastello and Adriano Sturli, added a fourth type a few years later.

Blood's Reciprocal Ingredients

Landsteiner found that there were two distinct agglutinogens, substances on the surfaces of red blood cells, that were responsible for clumping. He called them A and B. Based on the possible combinations of these agglutinogens, he labeled four types of human blood A, B, AB and O (which was neither A nor B). By one of nature's reciprocal arrangements, he realized, there were antagonistic substances in the plasma of each blood type that reacted violently with foreign red cells. Type A blood had anti-B agglutinin in its plasma; B had anti-A; AB had neither; and O had both anti-A and anti-B.

Therefore, B-type blood clumped A; and A clumped B. O was the universal donor; any blood type could receive it for transfusion. AB was the universal recipient. The reserved Landsteiner first mentioned his findings in a footnote to an article on blood variations within animal species: "The blood of some human beings destroys the red cells of other human beings." But it was not until eight years later in 1908 that the first transfusion was given under the safe conditions Landsteiner made possible. In New York, Reuben Ottenberg transfused tested, typed blood. There were no clumps of red blood cells clogging capillaries, no unexplained deaths, no mysterious reactions.

Typing blood by Landsteiner's system, now widely known as the ABO system, is still the most important step in matching individuals for safe transfusions. But hematologists have found, and continue to find, further idiosyncracies in the liquid tissue. There is every indication, re-

Karl Landsteiner

The Families of Blood

One spring day in 1880, when twelve-year-old Karl Landsteiner was walking home from a piano lesson, he collided with a bearded man on a Vienna sidewalk. The man wore the ribbon of the French Legion of Honor in his buttonhole and dragged his left leg in a limp. His cane clattered to the pavement as Landsteiner bumped into him, and the youth apologized for his carelessness. Later, he saw a picture of the man in the evening newspaper. He was the distinguished French scientist Louis Pasteur, in Vienna for a conference on cholera. As a boy, Landsteiner planned to be a musician. When he won his own Legion of Honor ribbon thirty years later, however, it was not as a celebrated pianist but as the virtuoso discoverer of human blood groups.

After graduating from medical school in 1891, Landsteiner became interested in blood transfusions. He heard surgeons complain that despite successful operations, their patients often died from blood loss. In America and Russia, some doctors were experimenting with transfusions but with limited success. Some patients recovered, but others died suddenly as if the blood transfused into their veins were poison.

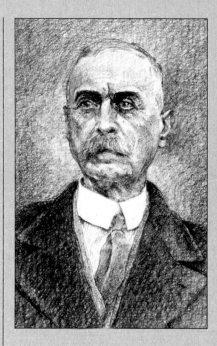

Intrigued by this medical mystery, Landsteiner began experimenting with blood serum. Commencing his studies with animals, he mixed the serum of one rabbit with the whole blood of another, observing no untoward reactions. He then mixed the serum of the second rabbit with the blood of the first and again noticed nothing unusual. But when Landsteiner combined rabbit serum with guinea pig blood, the mixture became a pool of yellow liquid, streaked with clumps of blood. The same reaction occurred when he blended human blood with animal serum.

It soon became evident to Landsteiner that the blood of different species was incompatible. When he intensified his research on human blood, he made another novel discovery. Although the blood of different people often mixed evenly, sometimes the red blood cells clumped, as though they came from different animals. Landsteiner reported his unusual findings on animal blood in a scholarly article published in 1900.

After months of research, he realized that the clumping of human red blood cells could not be a random occurrence. He and his researchers identified four major human blood groups, known today as A, B, AB and O. In later years, he helped identify another blood peculiarity that thwarted successful transfusions — the Rh factor. Despite the importance of Landsteiner's discovery, ten years passed before a doctor transfused blood using his safe, predictable methods. It took twenty years more before Landsteiner, by then a United States citizen, won a Nobel Prize. By 1930, however, the Swedish judges had merely confirmed what the world already knew, that the discovery of human blood groups was one of history's greatest medical achievements.

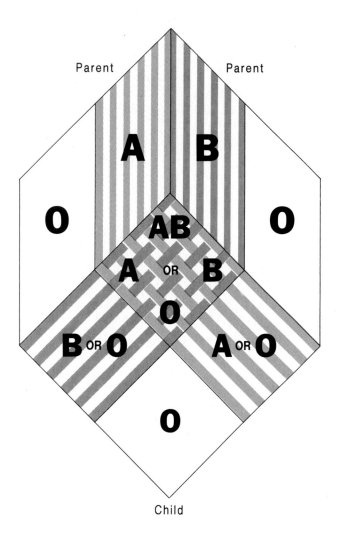

Parent   Parent

A   B
O   O
AB
A OR B
O
B OR O   A OR O
O

Child

This schematic diagram demon-strates how blood types are geneti-cally passed from parents to a child. Match any two blood types in the top row and follow the columns to their intersection.

searchers now think, that human blood may prove to be just as unique as human fingerprints.

Some forty years after he devised the ABO system, Landsteiner discovered another determinant in human blood — the Rh factor. This factor can be easily tested. When the blood of a rhesus monkey is injected into a rabbit, the rabbit's immune system develops antibodies. Then, when a sample of the rabbit's plasma is mixed with a sample of human red blood cells, the human cells will generally clump. Those who have blood that does clump are said to be Rh (from the monkey) positive. Those who have blood that does not clump have a negative Rh factor. About 85 percent of Americans have Rh positive blood.

The child of an Rh positive man and an Rh negative woman will have a 50 percent chance of being either. If an Rh negative mother carries an Rh positive baby, some of the baby's blood may diffuse through the placenta into the mother's blood stream. The mother's immune system can then produce potent antibodies against the alien Rh factor. If the next or any subsequent child is Rh positive, these antibodies can enter the embryo's blood, attack its red blood cells and kill the fetus. Scientists are still not sure why the first child is protected from the mother's antibodies.

Bloodprints of Life

Today, there are several hundred identifiable elements in red blood cells that contribute to a person's "bloodprint." Law courts in most states accept blood typing as solid evidence in crimes. Blood types can also be used to settle cases of paternity. Until recently, blood tests were usually used to prove that a man had not fathered a child, but the more costly process of typing to prove paternity has also been used for evidence. If the child and alleged father have five rare factors in common, factors that are not found in the mother, paternity can be proved. "Outside the family of the accused," claim hematologists Robert Race and Ruth Sanger, "there would not be another such man in ten million." A more recently developed test examines the white blood cells. Called H. L. A. (human leukocyte antigen), the test can accurately match white blood cell substances of the child with those of the father.

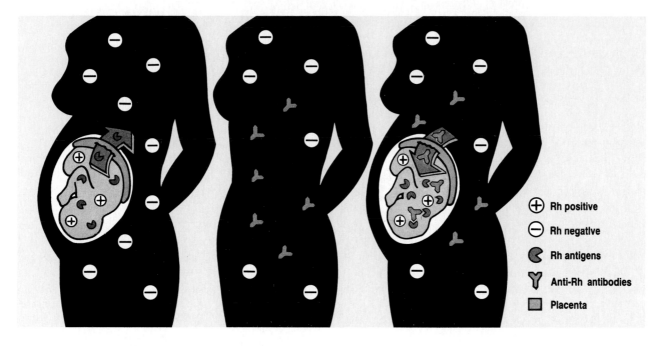

⊕ Rh positive

⊖ Rh negative

  Rh antigens

Y Anti-Rh antibodies

▮ Placenta

An unusual application of blood typing occurred in Austria in 1979. In this case, it was used to prove maternity. An AB-type mother, who, by the rules of genetic coding can have only A, B, or AB-type children, gave birth to a type O child. It was her fourth. Specialists examined genetic markings of the newborn and the other children and found traits that could not have been inherited from either parent. They did, however, find the traits in the mother's parents. It was as though the grandparents had passed on genetic characteristics that had somehow skipped a generation. Scientists theorize that the mother, when she was conceived in her mother's womb, was originally two fertilized eggs, each with different genes. Rather than developing into twins, these two eggs merged to form one fetus. One of the egg cells determined the mother's blood and her physical characteristics, and the other determined her egg cells. In effect, the mother was a pair of nonidentical twins.

So well understood are the genetics of blood group inheritance that typing has given anthropologists an invaluable tool for studying the races and migrations of man. The blood type of an individual is a constant that does not change with age or diet. Requiring only a drop of blood, it is also a relatively simple method of gathering genetic data. Blood typing has presented some intriguing puzzles to anthropological thought.

The people of central China have a high incidence of type B blood — about 35 percent. By tracing the geographical route their ancestors are thought to have followed from Asia across North and South America — the Bering Strait — researchers have discovered that the percentage of type B steadily decreases. Ten percent of Alaskan and Canadian Eskimos have type B blood; and 5 percent of the Indians of Central and South America have it; but for some reason, no Indians in the United States have type B.

More puzzling, all Indians in the Western hemisphere have a blood factor called Diego. It is a rare ingredient, but also found in 10 percent of the people of China and Japan. Anthropologists believe this might confirm a Mongol origin for Indians. Yet, no Eskimos have the Diego factor. "Strange is it," wrote Shakespeare, "that our bloods, of color, weight and heat, pour'd all together, would quite confound distinction, yet stands off in differences so mighty."

With the dream of sharing blood realized, the challenge remained to extend the gift. The great world wars were catalysts for developing new

Max Perutz

Mapping the Hemoglobin Molecule

Reflecting on his epic search for the molecular structure of hemoglobin, the complex protein in red blood cells that delivers oxygen to the tissues, Max Perutz said that he had often longed for an "elegant solution" to his quest. But, for twenty-five years, he found endless hours of hard work, rigorous measurement and exhausting calculation. The undertaking proved to be among the most difficult in modern science.

When Perutz first arrived at Cambridge University in 1936 to study, he believed that "the riddle of life was hidden in the structure of proteins." The following year, he chose to study hemoglobin, hardly expecting to spend his entire career unraveling its secrets. Since the 1860s, scientists had been aware that hemoglobin carried oxygen in the blood stream, and an English physiologist had calculated in the 1920s that a single hemoglobin molecule weighed 67,000 times more than a hydrogen atom. Of the architecture of the molecule, however, scientists knew virtually nothing.

To address the problem, Perutz used X-ray crystallography, a technique that reveals the hidden structure of crystals by beaming X-rays through them. Hemoglobin

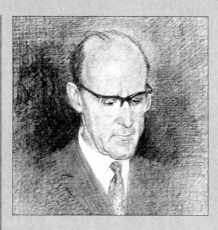

forms angular, garnet-colored crystals under certain conditions, making it well-suited for X-ray crystallography. Perutz and his colleagues took thousands of X-ray photographs of hemoglobin crystals from many angles, subjecting each plate to mathematical analysis.

At the beginning of World War II, Perutz's studies were interrupted when British authorities briefly imprisoned him in Quebec City because he was a native of Austria. After his release in 1941, he worked on a secret allied project to transform icebergs into floating landing strips for airplanes flying between England and the United States.

In 1945, Perutz resumed his work on hemoglobin. A major breakthrough came in 1951, when he learned how to attach mercury atoms to hemoglobin through chemical reactions.

Perutz called the discovery "the most exciting in all my research career." Knowing the position of the mercury atom on his X-ray plate allowed him to chart other atoms on the hemoglobin molecule.

Using complex mathematical methods, Perutz traced the structure of hemoglobin, achieving a three-dimensional understanding of the molecule in 1962. He found that one hemoglobin molecule held 10,000 atoms, locked together in four twisting chains. Each chain harbored a ring of carbon, nitrogen and hydrogen atoms, with an iron atom, like a jewel, at the center.

Another six years passed before Perutz transformed his calculations into a three-dimensional model of hemoglobin. Declaring that he had merely mapped the molecule's anatomy, he spent ten more years analyzing how hemoglobin worked. He discovered that one hemoglobin molecule carried only four oxygen molecules, loosely attached to the iron atoms, but it performed its task of delivering oxygen with near-perfect efficiency. As he neared the end of his quest, Perutz recalled the sensation of uncovering the interwoven structure of hemoglobin: "We felt like explorers who have discovered a new continent."

Clearly marked trails of evidence, blood types provide clues to the migrations of ancient man. In the map below, type B blood, which flows in 35 percent of the population of central China, diffuses westward through Europe, tracing the Mongol invasions of the thirteenth century. Moving eastward across the Bering Strait, type B blood also ties the North American Indians, including Inca and Eskimo, bottom, to common ancestry in Mongolia. Yet, Eskimos mysteriously lack the Diego factor — a more subtle genetic trait that links aboriginal Americans to Asia. Blood typing poses many such riddles for anthropologists.

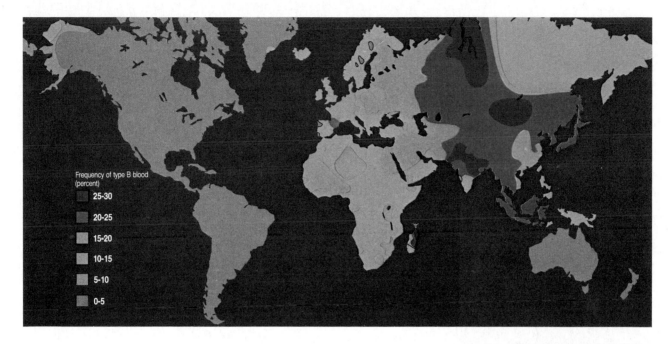

Frequency of type B blood
(percent)

- 25-30
- 20-25
- 15-20
- 10-15
- 5-10
- 0-5

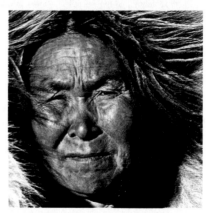

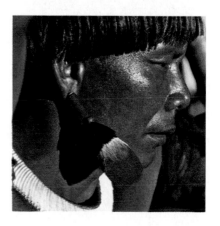

techniques for saving lives. O. H. Robertson, a Canadian medical officer during World War I, discovered that a solution of citrate glucose could preserve blood for as long as twenty-one days. The solution saved many shock victims. But, between the world wars, the idea of storing and transporting blood received little attention.

Bernard Fantus started the first blood bank in 1937 at the Cook County Hospital in Chicago. He found that blood treated with a 2 percent solution of sodium citrate would not clot and thus could be stored in refrigerators. But the blood never lasted more than ten days. Loaned at interest rates of 100 percent, each borrowed pint had to be replaced by two from the recipient when he recovered. This was a modest effort, only possible in a large hospital. By the time World War II broke out, transporting refrigerated blood to the front lines was as impractical as ever.

"In these times of war when men die on many fronts it becomes imperative to get either fresh or well-preserved blood to them or some substitute capable of sustaining fluid balance and circulation in the early hours of their injury." So wrote Charles Drew in 1939. He was a Ph. D. candidate at Columbia University, studying the feasibility of blood banking. The following year he reported

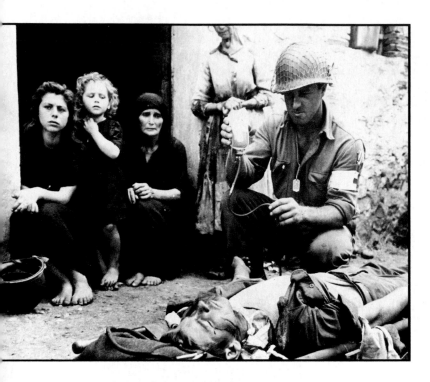

A French peasant family witnesses one of the first wartime transfusions, during World War II. A U.S. medic transfuses a soldier wounded in the liberation of France. Opposite, autotransfusion — recycling a patient's own blood — was an unsuccessful practice in the nineteenth century that recent technology now makes possible. Blood shed during surgery is collected, filtered, cleaned and returned to the patient. In some cases, the technique has reduced by as much as 60 percent the need for donated blood.

his findings to the National Blood Transfusion Committee, whose members were trying to solve the problem of transporting blood to occupied France. For cases of shock, burns and open wounds, plasma often worked better than whole blood, Drew told the members. It could also be stored and transported without refrigeration.

In the fall of 1940, the first plane carrying plasma left New York for besieged England. In the ensuing five months, 17,000 pints of American plasma helped save British lives — what some called the greatest experiment ever in brotherhood. England organized its own program based on the Blood for Britain project. As it seemed inevitable that America would join the war, the Blood Transfusion Committee and the American Red Cross formed a National Blood Bank program, headed by Drew. Their goal was to reserve one million pints of plasma, should the American military need it. On December 7, 1941, when the Japanese attacked Pearl Harbor, the reserve was put to use. Of every hundred wounded soldiers treated with plasma, ninety-six recovered.

Today almost 5 percent of all hospitalized patients receive blood transfusions, each averaging about three pints of blood. The techniques developed during wartime made the international network of blood sharing a reality. Organizations such as the American Association of Blood Banks (AABB) and the American Red Cross collect and distribute approximately eleven million pints of blood a year. More than 95 percent of this supply is given voluntarily; the rest is bought and sold commercially. Sophisticated computer systems can identify hundreds of rare blood types from all over the world and match donors to patients.

A transfusion technique once used in the nineteenth century has recently met with success and offers an alternative to transfusion and blood banking. Now known as intraoperative autotransfusion, it gives a person his own blood. Blood shed during surgery is not discarded; it is removed and cleaned, then put back in the body. Some hospitals use autotransfusion for all heart surgery, cutting by as much as 60 percent the need for donated blood in such operations. But, even better, patients receive the best kind of blood available — their own.

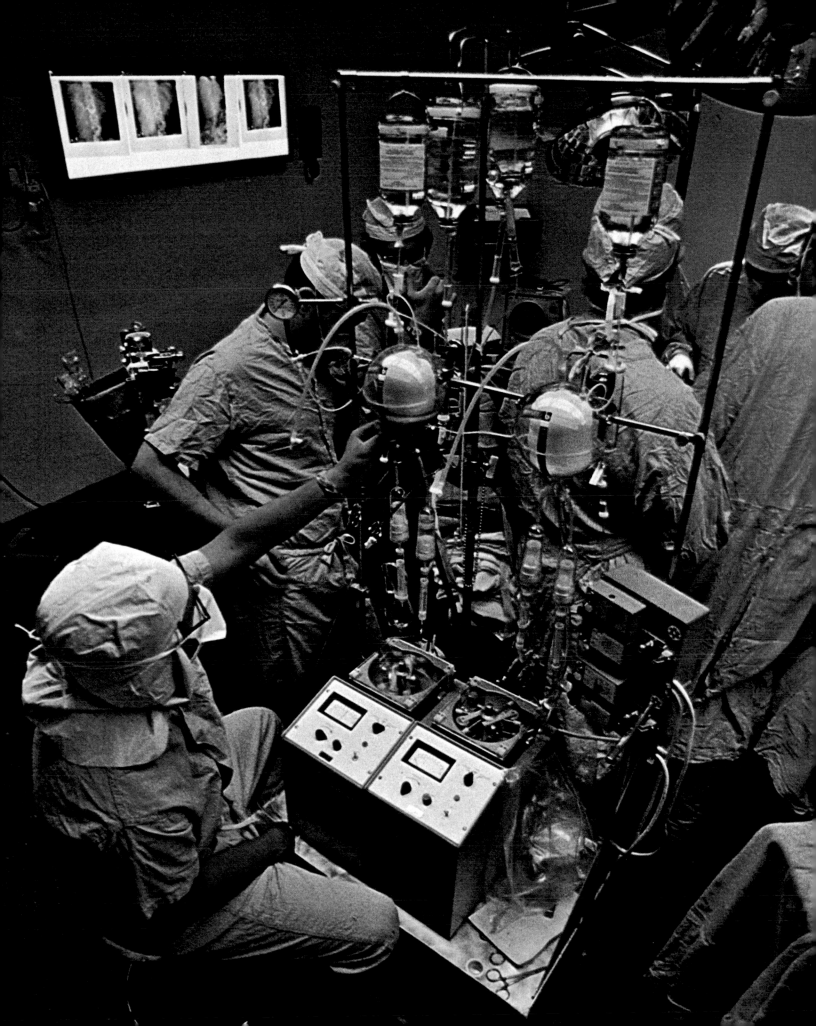

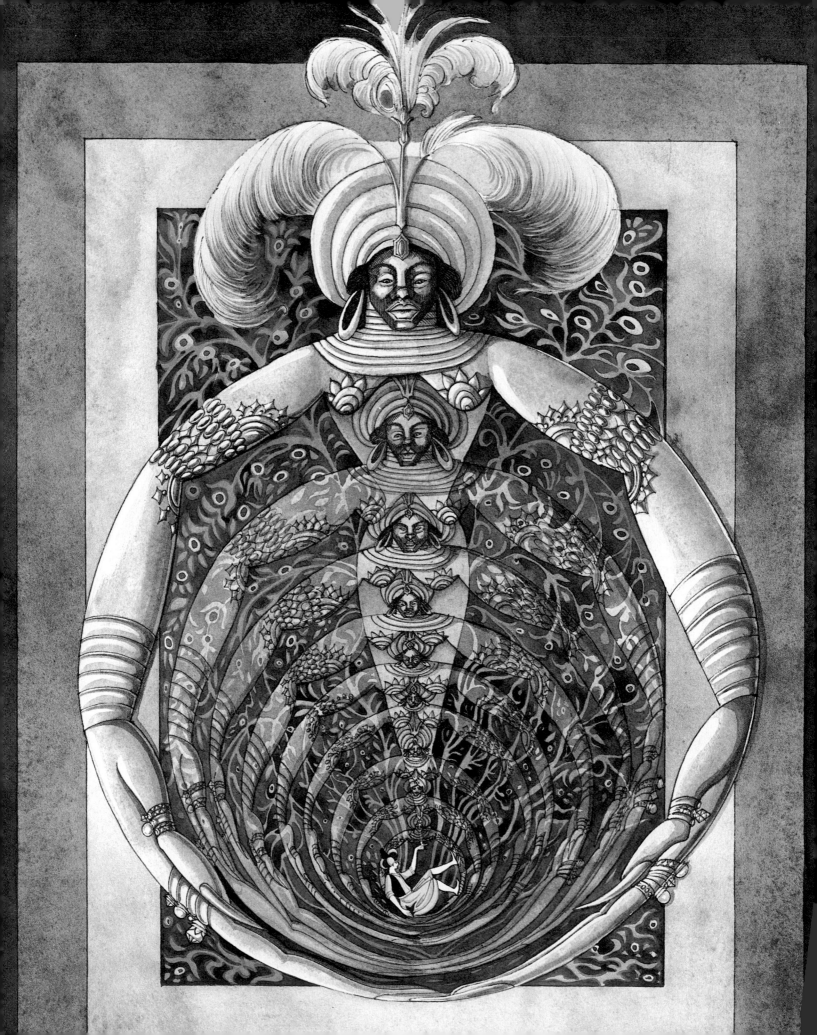

Chapter 3

The Great Exchange

Severed from its mother, cradled upside-down and patted on the back, the newborn infant draws its first breath. With a scream, the child empties its lungs to begin respiration, the perpetual exchange binding it to the world it will live in. Man's need for oxygen is relentless. He can live for days without water, weeks without food. But denied oxygen for just five minutes, his brain suffers lasting damage. A little longer and the glow of life fades to dusk. At the same time, carbon dioxide must be steadily expelled from the body. Blood, traveling from the lungs to the cells, carries out this ceaseless transaction. It gathers oxygen and releases carbon dioxide through the lungs, all the while unloading oxygen and collecting carbon dioxide at the cells. Breathing, in concert with heartbeat, marks time like a pair of drums, laying down steady rhythms against which other processes resound.

Blood is the atmosphere in which body cells live and breathe. About 60 percent of the weight of the human body is water. Roughly 40 percent of this is the fluid within the cells themselves. The rest, called extracellular fluid, is one part blood plasma and four parts interstitial fluid, the liquid between and around the cells. A sea within man, interstitial fluid swarms with the cells to which it gives life. The river of blood flows continually through this sea, nourishing, cleansing and balancing it.

The Vital Balance

Together, sea and river make up what Claude Bernard, celebrated French physiologist of the last century, called the *milieu intérieur*, the internal environment of the body. This must remain as stable as the external environment is changeable. Man enjoys so much choice over where and how he lives because his body demands so small a conscious part in maintaining the internal balances essential to life.

Aladdin, finding sanctuary within the enchanted embrace of the genie, casts off fear of perils stalking the world. Blood too traces charmed circles, safeguarding man within balanced rings of defenses against the extremes of his surroundings and the caprice of his nature.

Bound one with another, these balances strike an equilibrium known as homeostasis. W. B. Cannon, the physiologist who coined the word, called it "the wisdom of the body." Body temperature is perhaps the most familiar of the balances struck whether man be hot or cold, asleep or awake, hungry or slaked. Any change in the internal environment automatically spurs organs, tissues and cells to offset the change and restore the balance. Each cell, in its own distinctive way, contributes to the vitality of the body by maintaining the stability of the fluid bathing all cells. Blood is the medium through which balance is kept. Blood travels completely through the body once each minute, making two continuous circuits. On the first — the pulmonary circulation — blood loops from the heart through the lungs, turning from leaden blue to crimson, then returns to the heart. On the second — the systemic circulation — blood, laden with oxygen, travels to the far reaches of the body, shedding oxygen and gathering carbon dioxide, and once again returns it to the heart. In *The Rape of Lucrece*, Shakespeare followed blood's odyssey in rhyme:

> ... bubbling from her breast, it doth divide
> In two slow rivers, that the crimson blood
> Circles her body in one every side ...
> Some of her blood still pure and red remain'd
> And some look'd black ...

Pressure, originally imparted by the power of the heart, keeps blood moving against the friction of the increasingly smaller vessels through which it flows. Driven from the heart, blood rushes rapidly from larger to smaller arteries, where, losing pace and pressure, it enters the arterioles. Arterioles control the flow of blood to the tissues. One arteriole can serve a hundred capillaries. Strong muscular walls bristling with nerve fibers enable an arteriole to close or expand. From the arterioles, blood trickles through still narrower vessels, the metarterioles. Passing a muscular valve called the precapillary sphincter, blood passes next into the tiny vessels called capillaries. Like latticework, capillaries are woven throughout tissues. Blood enters capillaries from arterioles and leaves through venules which join to veins. Capillaries deliver nutrients to cells and

The cells making up the human body live in conditions as fixed as those outside the body are changeable. Blood binds the internal environment of the body to the world outside, maintaining the constancy of the first against changes in the second. Pumped by the heart, blood rises to the lungs, collecting oxygen from the atmosphere. Filled with oxygen, blood returns to the heart, then courses throughout the body. In the intestines, blood gathers food particles, then takes them to the liver. Here, man's diet is transformed into the chemical diet of cells. Taken from the world beyond the body to cells within it, oxygen and food combine to produce energy. Just as blood delivers nourishment, so does it remove waste. The kidneys constantly refine blood, preserving its chemical balance while expelling waste. Once more returning to the heart and looping to the lungs, blood releases carbon dioxide as it collects oxygen before circling the body again. Blood enables all the organs to play as an ensemble, striking the balance which the internal environment requires. Scientists call this balance homeostasis — the balance of nature in man.

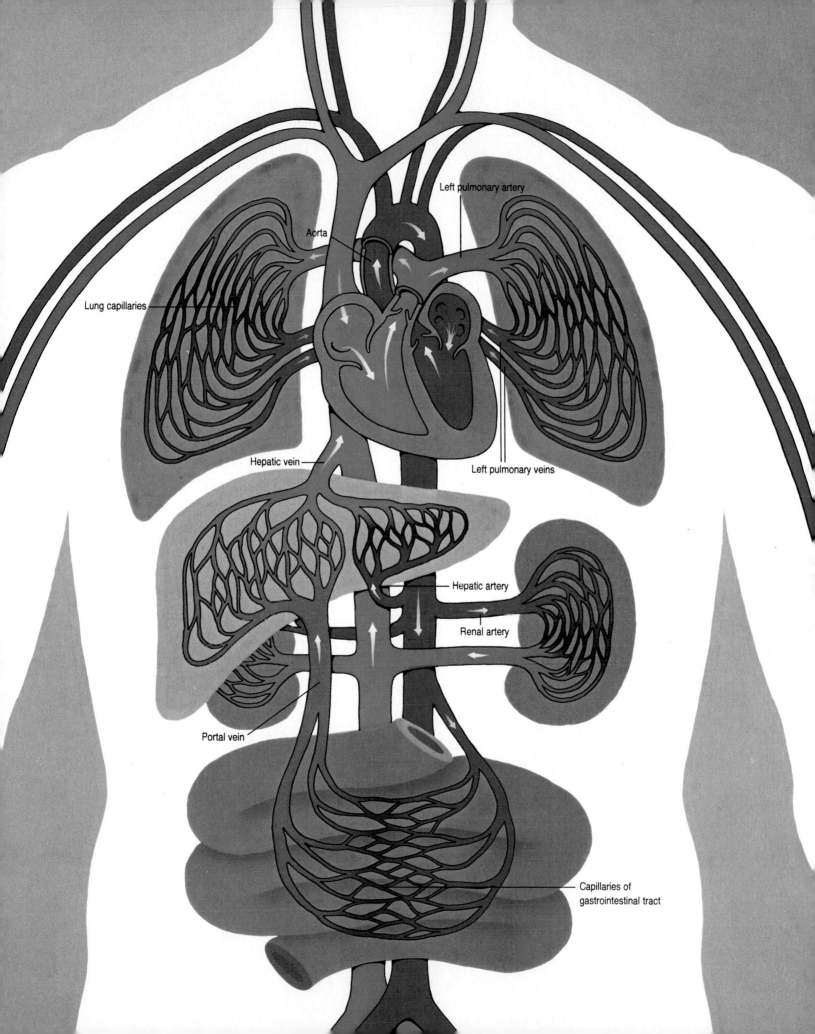

collect waste from them. At the venous end of the capillary, blood begins its return to the heart, completing the systemic circulation.

The flow of blood to the tissues is controlled by the brain, adrenal glands, kidneys and the tissues themselves. Responding to different signals carried by the blood, the arterioles, metarterioles and precapillary sphincters stanch or free blood into the capillaries. Tissues control blood flow by adjusting it to their need for nutrients like oxygen, sugars and acids. How tissues exercise this control is not clear. Some researchers suggest that when short of nutrients, tissues manufacture substances that cause the precapillary sphincter, metarterioles and arterioles to dilate, and so increase blood flow. Others think lack of nutrients alone causes dilation. Most agree that because different tissues perform different functions and have different needs, both processes operate.

Three other processes, originating in the brain, the adrenal glands and the kidneys, augment the tissues' control of blood flow, particularly during injury. Arteries and arterioles, as well as veins and venules, contain nerve fibers linking them to the vasomotor center, the part of the brain that affects blood vessels. The vasomotor center signals these nerve fibers to secrete norepinephrine, a vasoconstrictor agent that stimulates blood vessels to contract. The nervous system can override demands of tissues as it distributes blood by acting locally on particular vessels. But the adrenal glands, perched atop the kidneys, also secrete norepinephrine, as well as another vasoconstrictor, epinephrine, into the blood stream. The kidneys secrete renin, an enzyme that triggers a series of reactions leading to the production of angiotensin, a powerful vasoconstrictor. Serious injury accompanied by profuse bleeding can drive blood pressure dangerously low. In response, the brain produces and secretes the strongest of the vasoconstrictor agents, vasopressin. Circulating throughout the body, vasoconstrictors act rapidly on all blood vessels except capillaries. These substances regulate the flow of blood even in vessels beyond the reach of the nervous system.

All three systems for regulating the control and distribution of blood flow require that pressure

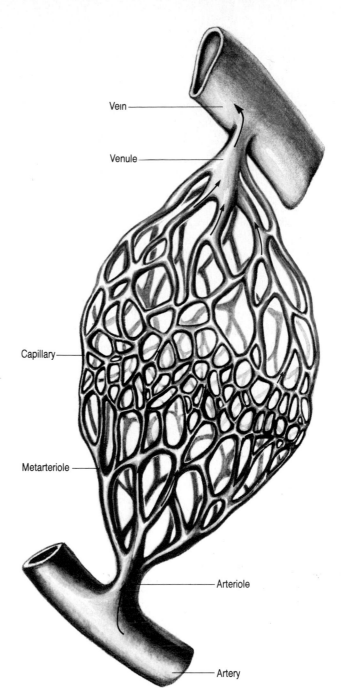

Blood begins its return to the heart in capillaries, above, changing from red to blue. For centuries, inquirers tracking cirulation lost it in thickets of these tiny vessels. Finally, in 1661, Italian anatomist Marcello Malpighi discovered that capillaries linked veins and arteries. Fanning out like fronds of a fern, capillaries, opposite, shade all body tissues in blood. Arterioles branch at right angles from an artery to send out metarterioles into beds of capillaries.

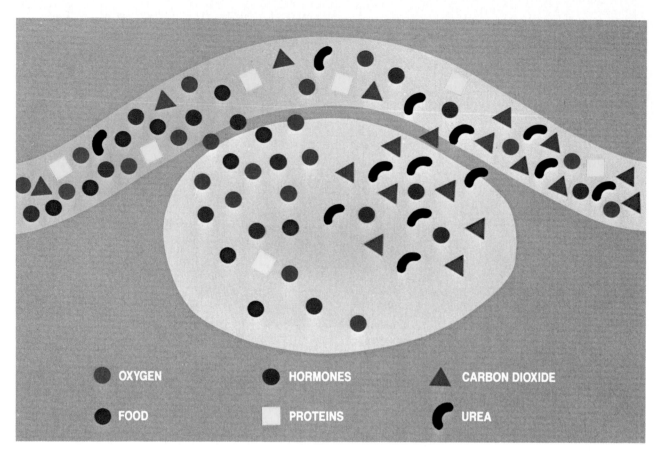

| ● OXYGEN | ● HORMONES | ▲ CARBON DIOXIDE |
| ● FOOD | ■ PROTEINS | ◗ UREA |

in the arterial vessels remain constant. Otherwise, constriction or dilation of the vessels would not necessarily decrease or increase local blood flow. Vasoconstrictor agents help regulate arterial pressure as they course through the blood stream. But the chief regulators of arterial pressure are baroreceptors. These splayed nerve endings are found in nearly every artery but are most numerous in the carotid artery in the neck, the chief vessel feeding the brain, and the aortic arch, where arteries stemming from the heart begin their descent into the lower body. When blood volume in an artery shrinks or swells, lowering or raising pressure, baroreceptors alert the brain. The brain, in turn, tenses or relaxes vessels, returning blood pressure to normal. When, after lying down, a person suddenly sits or stands up, blood pressure plummets. The brain and the baroreceptors adjust pressure so quickly that only rarely does light-headedness result. Vasoconstrictor substances and baroreceptor reflexes regulate pressure second by second. By this coordinated means of monitoring flow and pressure, blood ultimately flows to the capillaries.

Here, in a split second, only 5 percent of the circulating blood performs the great exchange. Some ten billion capillaries lace all body tissues,

bringing blood to within easy reach of every cell. Because capillary walls are but one cell thick, they are highly permeable. To reach cells, substances in the blood must first pass through the capillary wall into the interstitial fluid surrounding the cell. Waste produced by the cells makes the same passage into capillaries, only in reverse.

Most substances freely cross the capillary walls by a process known as diffusion: Fueled by their own heat, molecules in blood are in constant, random motion. If the blood is divided by a permeable barrier, like a capillary wall or cell membrane, the molecules will break the barrier from where they are most concentrated to where they are least concentrated. Blood in a capillary has a higher concentration of oxygen than does interstitial fluid. The difference in concentration, known as the diffusion gradient, causes oxygen to pass through the capillary wall into the interstitial fluid. Likewise, when interstitial fluid has a higher concentration of carbon dioxide than capillary blood, the diffusion gradient causes carbon dioxide to move from the interstitial fluid across the capillary wall into the blood.

Even distribution of fluid is crucial to homeostasis. Opposing pressures in the blood and the interstitium distribute fluids evenly between the

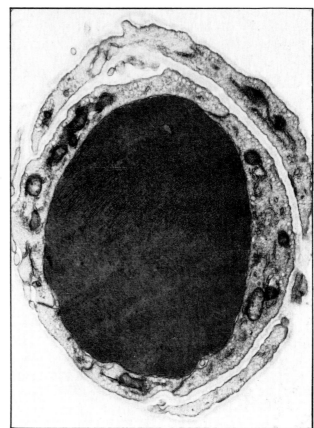

two. When capillary walls are damaged by a sharp blow, the balance of pressures is upset. Fluid leaks out of capillaries, flooding the interstitium. This condition, known as edema, is experienced as blisters or swelling.

To complete the great exchange of oxygen and carbon dioxide, substances must pass back and forth between the interstitium and the cell. Life springs ultimately from the activity of cells as they consume and produce the substances carried by the blood. Fully 24 percent of body weight, fluid within the cells has a very different chemical composition from extracellular fluid. Extracellular fluid is rich in sodium and chloride but poor in potassium. Inside the cell, these proportions are reversed. Magnesium, abundant inside cells, is scarce outside them. Phosphates and proteins are both more plentiful in the intracellular fluid. Their arrangement arises from exchanges between cells and blood via the interstitial fluid.

Just as substances must cross the capillary wall, so must they cross the cell membrane. A thin elastic film enclosing the cell, the membrane is made up of lipids, substances which easily dissolve in fats. Suspended in the lipids are protein particles. Nutrients breach the membrane in one of two ways: diffusion or active transport.

Capillaries carry blood laden with nutrients to cells. Like a barge moored alongside a quay, a cell and a capillary swap cargoes, opposite. Oxygen, carbon dioxide and foodstuffs are their staples of trade. Hormones are also exchanged. Plasma proteins remain in the blood stream, while urea is taken from cells like bilge. Bristling beneath the skin, the capillaries, above left, lace a fingertip, bringing blood to enliven the stroke of a cheek, the twist of a tool or the pluck of a lyre. A cross section of a single capillary, above, magnified 20,000 times, reveals its thin, permeable wall. Substances pass easily back and forth across capillary walls. When wear and tear damages capillaries, fluids spill out across the walls, causing blisters and swelling.

Different substances diffuse through the membrane in different ways and at different rates. Oxygen, carbon dioxide, alcohol and fatty acids dissolve in the lipids of the membrane and cross freely, as they would through a capillary wall. Other substances, notably glucose and amino acids, do not dissolve in lipids but combine with a carrier, a substance that is lipid-soluble. The carrier escorts them across the membrane by a process called facilitated diffusion. Other substances such as water and dissolved minerals seem to slip through pores in the membrane.

Substances always diffuse from high to low concentrations, and with, never against, a diffusion gradient. But potassium, required by all cells, is sparsely concentrated in extracellular fluid. Sodium on the other hand, is much richer outside the cells from which it must be removed. These substances cross the cell membrane, against diffusion gradients, with the help of a carrier by active transport. This is similar to diffusion, except that in this process, the carrier moves its consort against the diffusion gradient.

More a filter than a frontier, the cell membrane admits and expels diverse substances in balanced amounts at appropriate rates, maintaining the subtle chemical balances on which cells depend.

Tending Life's Fires

Ceaselessly coursing through the body and among the cells, blood diligently stokes and tends the fires of life. Life arises from energy generated by cells, energy released when oxygen combines with other nutrients in what scientists call oxidation. To the cells, blood brings both food and the oxygen needed to burn it. At the same time, blood takes away the fumes and ashes from these perpetual fires. The fires of independent life are kindled at birth when the newborn draws its first breath.

At rest, man draws about a dozen breaths every minute, taking in fresh atmospheric air. About one-fifth of this air fills the dead space of the respiratory passages in the throat and chest, never reaching the lungs. He exhales an equal amount of stale air. Yet the lungs are never empty. At any one moment they hold nearly five times the amount of air drawn in with each breath. It takes more than sixteen breaths to completely renew the air in the lungs.

From the nose or mouth, air travels down the windpipe. This channel divides into the bronchi, two tubes, one leading to each lung. Inside the lungs the bronchi send off shoot after shoot of wispy tubes. These are the bronchioles. At the end of each bronchiole, like clusters of grapes on vines, are tiny air sacs, the alveoli. Some 300 million alveoli fill the two lungs, giving them their characteristic spongy texture. Like climbing tendrils, the pulmonary arterioles and venules wind their way along the bronchioles, then branch out to form dense webs of capillaries entwining the alveoli. Enveloped by a thin film of water, the alveoli and their capillaries together make up the respiratory membrane. Laid flat, the respiratory membrane would carpet a room thirty feet long and twenty-five feet wide. At any one time, the capillaries hold just three ounces of blood. So little blood spread so thinly makes it possible for oxygen and carbon dioxide to be exchanged in just a quarter of a second.

The exchange begins when air, drawn into the alveoli from the atmosphere, and blood, rising into the capillaries from the heart, meet along the respiratory membrane. The air in the lungs is a mixture of gases — oxygen, carbon dioxide, nitrogen and water vapor. Like any gaseous mixture, this air is pressurized. Pressure is measured by the height to which the mixture can raise a column of mercury, expressed as millimeters of mercury, or mm. Hg. The pressure of each gas in the mixture, measured separately, is called its partial pressure. Differences in the partial pressures of oxygen and carbon dioxide along the respiratory membrane bring about diffusion. Oxygen, under higher partial pressure in the alveoli than in the capillaries, diffuses from the lungs into the blood. At the same time, carbon dioxide, under higher partial pressure in the capillaries than in the alveoli, diffuses from the blood into the lungs. Diffusion is continuous and rapid. But, since air in the alveoli is only slowly and gradually replaced, there are no sharp and sudden changes in the concentrations of gases.

In times of exertion or exercise, an individual may need fifteen to twenty times more oxygen

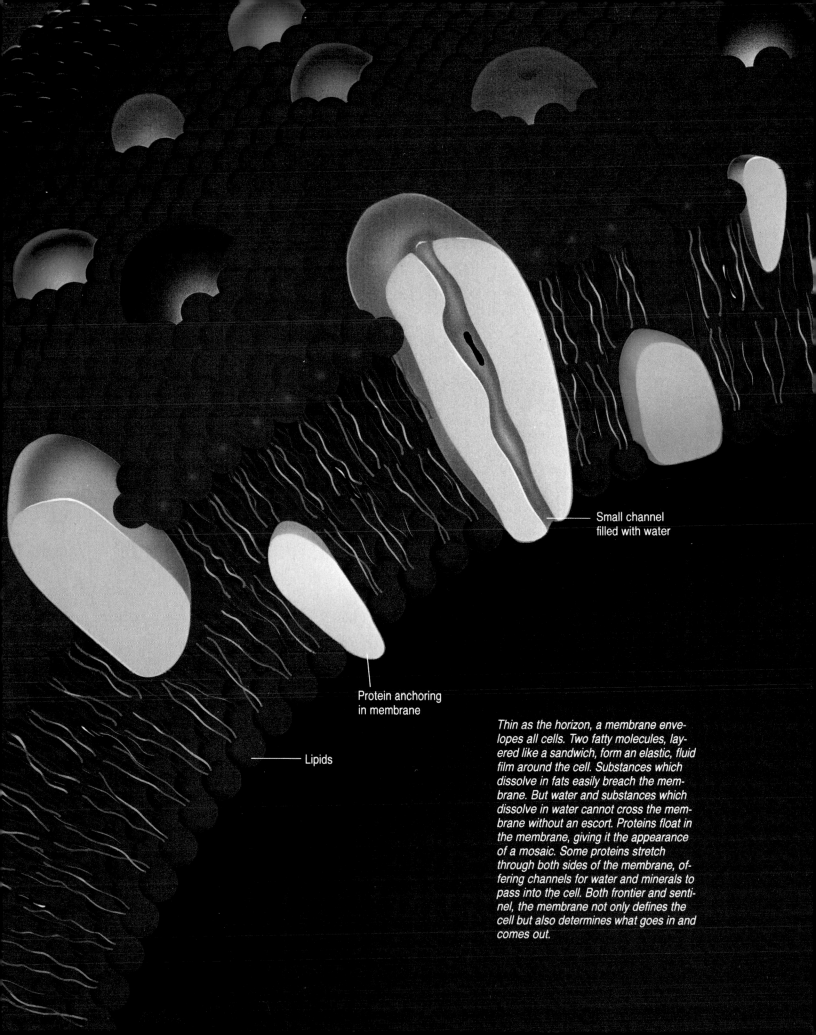

Small channel
filled with water

Protein anchoring
in membrane

Lipids

Thin as the horizon, a membrane enve-
lopes all cells. Two fatty molecules, lay-
ered like a sandwich, form an elastic, fluid
film around the cell. Substances which
dissolve in fats easily breach the membrane. But water and substances which
dissolve in water cannot cross the membrane without an escort. Proteins float in
the membrane, giving it the appearance
of a mosaic. Some proteins stretch
through both sides of the membrane, offering channels for water and minerals to
pass into the cell. Both frontier and senti-
nel, the membrane not only defines the
cell but also determines what goes in and
comes out.

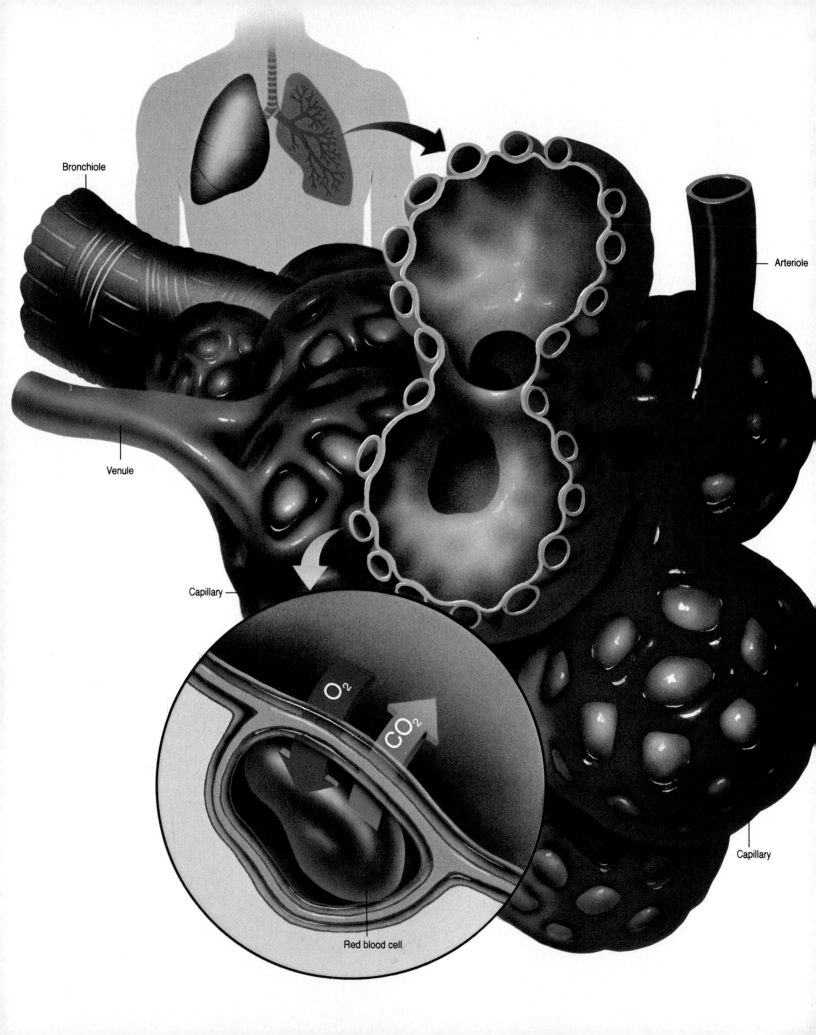

Bronchiole

Venule

Capillary

Arteriole

Capillary

O² CO²

Red blood cell

*Bellows within bellows, alveoli,
small as pinpoints, capture oxygen
and release carbon dioxide. Red
blood cells, inching along capillaries
in single file, swap carbon dioxide
for the oxygen they deliver to cells.*

than he needs at rest. The heart pumps blood through the pulmonary capillaries twice as fast as usual. Although blood requires more oxygen during exertion, it has less time to collect it. Still, it obtains nearly all the oxygen it can carry because more alveoli and capillaries are called to action. Diffusion of oxygen increases nearly threefold. These automatic processes ensure that during times of increased flow, enough oxygen meets the greater demands of tissues.

The Reliable Carrier

Passing into the blood, oxygen binds at once with hemoglobin in red blood cells, forming oxyhemoglobin, for transport to tissues and cells. Hemoglobin enables blood to carry between thirty and one hundred times more oxygen than if the oxygen were transported as a dissolved gas in the blood stream. The extent to which oxygen binds with hemoglobin is also determined by the partial pressure of oxygen in the alveoli. The normal partial pressure of oxygen is 100 mm. Hg. But because of its unique affinity for oxygen, hemoglobin binds 90 percent of the oxygen it can carry at a pressure of only 60 mm. Hg. Higher pressures of oxygen cause only slight increases in the amount of oxygen carried by hemoglobin. Likewise, when the partial pressure in tissue capillaries of oxygen falls, hemoglobin releases oxygen. Thus, the collection and release of oxygen depend on its partial pressure in the pulmonary and tissue capillaries.

When a person climbs a mountain or swims deep in the sea, the partial pressure of oxygen in his lungs may fall by half or rise fivefold. How, in the thin air on mountain tops, does he get the oxygen he needs? At 10,000 feet, the partial pressure of oxygen in the lungs falls to 60 mm. Hg. But even at this pressure, hemoglobin collects 90 percent of the oxygen it can carry, ensuring that tissues get enough oxygen. When a person swims underwater at a depth of 33 feet, the partial pressure of oxygen in the lungs rises to about 500 mm. Hg. But, since hemoglobin is nearly fully laden with oxygen at a pressure of 104 mm. Hg., oxygen in the blood increases only slightly, despite the sharp rise in pressure. Only when he climbs higher or dives deeper does he need me-

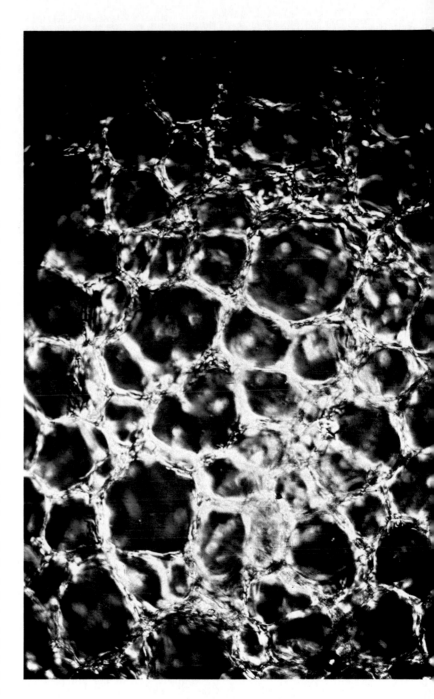

Flattened out, alveoli, ringed by capillaries, resemble cloisonné, the fine enamelware crafted since antiquity. The surface area of the alveoli in the lungs, if spread out, would cover 1,210 pages the size of this one.

Claude Bernard

Explorer of the *Milieu Intérieur*

"The science of life," French scientist Claude Bernard said, "is a superb and dazzlingly lighted hall which may be reached only by passing through a long and ghastly kitchen." At the intellectual feast of nineteenth century science, few toiled harder than Bernard himself, and few did more to illuminate the splendid hall. Despite the drudgery, his was a labor of love, for he also proclaimed that "the joy of discovery . . . is certainly the liveliest that any man can feel."

Growing up in a small village near Lyons, Bernard originally planned to become a playwright, spending his spare time composing poetry and drama. In 1834, at the age of twenty-one, he traveled to Paris to show the manuscript of a five-act play to St. Marc Girardin, a celebrated critic. Although Girardin recognized Bernard's talent, he counseled him to study medicine, saying that it would "much more surely gain you a livelihood."

Bernard dropped his literary ambitions and entered medical school. After graduating, he worked as a research assistant with François Magendie, the leading physiologist in France. In time, however, Bernard greatly outshone his mentor. He was the first to deduce the

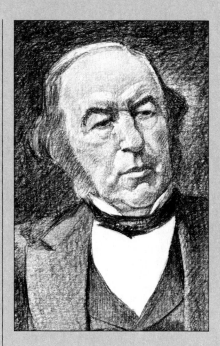

intestine's role in digestion, as well as the importance of the pancreas in breaking down fat. He also advanced a sophisticated theory of the body as a self-regulating mechanism, an idea followed in modern medicine. Bernard conceived of the inner world of the body, which he called the *milieu intérieur*, as a wholly different environment from the larger outside world, with different rules governing its operations.

He arrived at this notion partly through his research on blood. While studying heat regulation in the body, he cut a nerve in a rabbit's neck and saw that one side of the

rabbit's head became warmer. Bernard then proved that the nerve expanded or constricted the arteries leading to the head. On hot days, when blood must be cooled, the nerve causes the arteries to expand as they carry warm blood away from the head. On cold days, when heat must be conserved, the nerve tightens the arteries.

In another major discovery, Bernard revealed the lethal mechanism of carbon monoxide. Since ancient times, it was known that gases from charcoal fires were poisonous. Bernard demonstrated that carbon monoxide deprived the body of oxygen by combining with hemoglobin, the normal vehicle for carrying oxygen to the tissues. Thus, he found that poisoning from carbon monoxide causes an insidious form of asphyxiation.

For his many achievements, Bernard was elected to the French Academy, and upon his death in 1878 he became the first French scientist accorded a state funeral. In spite of his success, however, he remained humbled by the mysteries of nature, declaring, "Our feelings lead us at first to believe that absolute truth must lie within our realm; but study takes from us, little by little, these chimerical conceits."

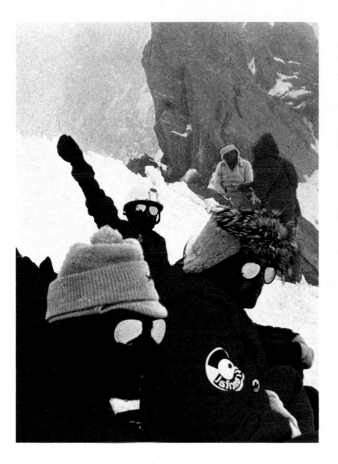

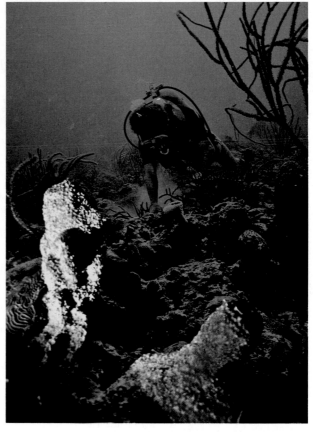

chanical devices to help him breathe. Otherwise, hemoglobin carries neither too little nor too much oxygen, and body tissues obtain sufficient oxygen despite extremes of pressure at the lungs.

At the tissue capillaries, the exchange ends. Oxygen diffuses across capillary walls through the interstitial fluid to the cells. At the same time, carbon dioxide from the cells enters the blood stream by the opposite route. Small amounts of carbon dioxide simply dissolve in the blood which transports it to the lungs, where it then is expelled. Some of it enters the lungs bound with hemoglobin. But roughly 70 percent undergoes a chain of chemical reactions which helps to maintain the acid-base balance in the body.

Acids and bases can be very powerful. Acids are used to refine uranium, the heaviest natural metal. Lye, a common base, is found in household cleansers. The body constantly consumes and produces both acids and bases. Chemically,

High in the Himalayas, air is thin and oxygen scarce. Even so, these Nepalese mountaineers, resting on the slopes of the world's second highest peak, get enough oxygen. Their bodies produce more red blood cells to capture as much of the sparse oxygen as possible. Each red cell carries nearly all the oxygen it can. Only at the roof of the world will climbers don oxygen masks. Beneath the sea, air pressure mounts rapidly. Prowling a reef, a diver risks getting too much oxygen. But his red blood cells, nearly laden with oxygen at sea level pressure, do not deliver more oxygen than his body can handle. Blood's transport of oxygen enables man to live, work and play at all altitudes.

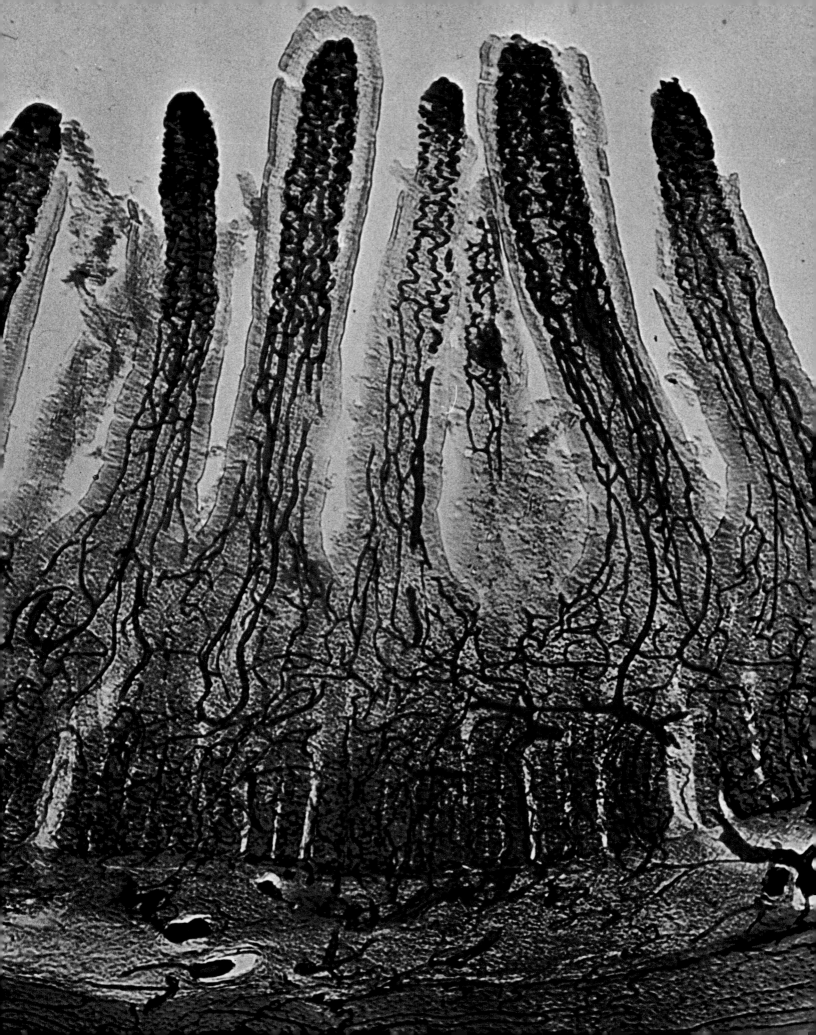

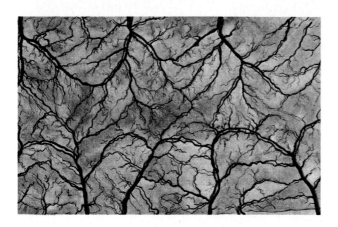

acids and bases are characterized by their concentrations of hydrogen ions. Water, consisting of two atoms of hydrogen and one of oxygen, has a slight tendency to break up so that part of a hydrogen atom goes astray. The stray part is a hydrogen ion. What remains — an oxygen atom, a hydrogen atom and the electron of the missing hydrogen ion — is a hydroxide ion. The reaction works both ways. After splitting up, some particles recombine to form water until equilibrium is reached. Water at equilibrium contains equal amounts of each ion, making it neutral.

The ions are balanced like a seesaw. Solutions turn acid when the concentration of their hydrogen ions rises, and turn basic when it falls. Chemists measure the concentration of hydrogen ions by pH, "p" standing for power and "H," for hydrogen ions. The pH of a neutral solution like water is 7.0. Low pH indicates an acid, high pH a base. Blood, with a normal pH of 7.4, is slightly basic. Because hydrogen ions are very active chemically, the presence of too many or too few will thwart the countless chemical reactions on which the body depends. The range within which the pH of blood can safely fluctuate is very narrow. It must not rise above 7.46 or fall below 7.32. Threatening so much and poised so finely, the acid-base balance is perhaps the most important aspect of homeostasis.

This balance is maintained by buffers, chemical partnerships which keep the pH constant by countering changes in the concentration of hydrogen ions. One buffer, called the bicarbonate buffer, arises from the transport of carbon dioxide by the blood. Not only does carbon dioxide dissolve in the water in blood, but it also reacts with water in red blood cells to form carbonic acid. Carbonic acid breaks down into hydrogen and bicarbonate ions. After releasing oxygen, hemoglobin binds with hydrogen ions and carries them to the lungs. As blood enters the pulmonary capillaries, these reactions reverse themselves. Hemoglobin binds with oxygen and releases hydrogen ions. Hydrogen and bicarbonate ions combine, forming carbonic acid. Then, carbonic acid breaks down to carbon dioxide and water. Finally the lungs expel carbon dioxide. Thus, in normal circumstances, respiration maintains pH by steadily expelling the carbon dioxide. Harnessed to breathing, the work of the bicarbonate buffer can adjust to the rate of respiration. After strenuous exercise or during severe shock, the concentration of hydrogen ions climbs sharply. Breathing quickens to flush out excess carbon dioxide, depleting the hydrogen ions and returning the pH to normal. Because this buffer works constantly, the amount of carbon dioxide in the blood, not the need for oxygen in the tissues, controls the rate of breathing.

Oxygen instead controls the flow of blood carrying the nutrients. Blood collects nutrients along the small intestine where food, passing through its twenty-three-foot length, is primarily broken down by the action of digestive juices. The walls of the small intestine are lined with a thick nap of fine pile made up of millions upon millions of tiny projections called villi. A network of capillaries, together with a lymph vessel, runs inside each tiny villus. Broken down by digestion into molecules, food and water pass from the intestinal canal into the blood stream at the villi by the process of absorption.

Digested food consists of components of carbohydrates, proteins and fats, each of which the blood stream handles differently. Carbohydrates, eaten mainly as starch from plants, are first broken into simple sugars. In the blood stream, these sugars are converted primarily to glucose, the fundamental fuel of cells. Unlike oxygen, which we inhale steadily, glucose enters the blood stream in varying amounts at sporadic intervals, depending on when and what we eat.

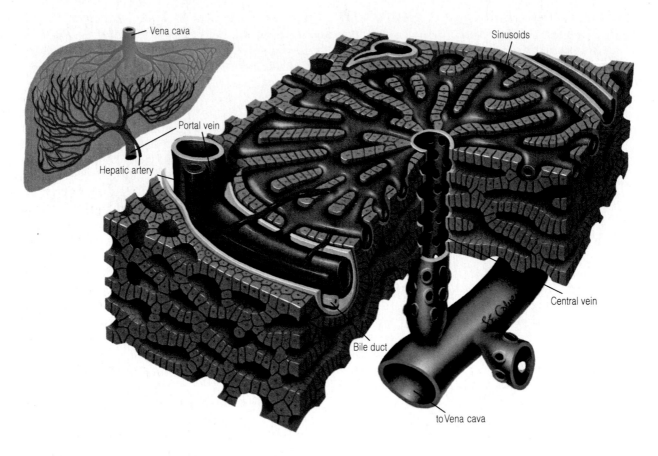

Vena cava

Sinusoids

Portal vein

Hepatic artery

Central vein

Bile duct

to Vena cava

How does the body manage to deliver a steady supply of glucose to the cells despite irregular eating habits? The liver releases glucose into the blood stream in regular quantities. Capillaries in the villi carry glucose to a large vessel, the portal vein, running from the intestines to the liver. The liver consists of between 50,000 and 100,000 lobules, tiny hexagonal units honeycombed with blood vessels. At the liver, the portal vein divides first into venules then into sinusoids — small, twisting vessels which lace the lobules. Apart from the blood carried by the portal vein, the liver, unlike any other organ, has a second source of blood, the hepatic artery. This blood first nourishes liver tissues, then mixes with blood from the portal vein, filling the sinusoids and soaking the lobules. Blood drains into the central veins of each lobule and flows from the liver through hepatic veins to the vena cava. Each minute some 30 percent of the blood pumped by the heart passes through the liver. After a meal, most glucose is removed from the blood by the liver, which uses a little, but stores the bulk. But glucose dissolves easily and cannot be stored without disrupting the work of liver cells. Thus, the liver converts glucose to glycogen, which does not dissolve and is easily stored. Between

meals, when there is little glucose in the blood, the liver converts glycogen back to glucose to be released into the blood stream through the hepatic vein. Once it leaves the liver, blood contains a balanced amount of glucose.

After digestion, proteins enter the blood stream as amino acids and pass into the liver through the portal vein. The liver puts amino acids to several uses, converting some into carbohydrates, fats or new chemical compounds, that form new amino acids. Still others are changed back into protein and returned to the blood in the form of plasma proteins — albumin, globulins and fibrinogen.

Fats must also undergo various changes before they can serve as nourishment. Some pass through the lymphatic system from the villi before reaching the blood stream. Yet others are taken to the liver which combines certain fats with proteins. The liver must always be awash with blood to perform its metabolic functions. Cirrhosis and other conditions which limit or restrict blood flow in the liver have profound consequences throughout the body.

Not all nutrients reaching the cells are digested. Minerals and water are absorbed directly into the blood stream, primarily at the small intestine,

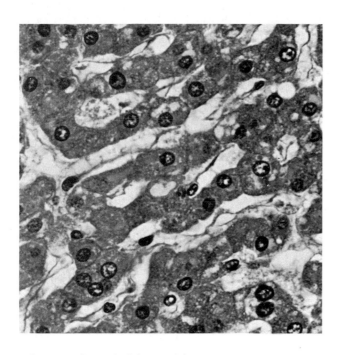

Like an enchanted alchemist, the liver takes digested food particles and turns them into the rich and varied diet body cells require. The liver, alone among organs, receives blood from two sources. Blood delivers food particles from the digestive tract to the liver through the portal vein, while the hepatic artery nourishes the liver with arterial blood. Shot through with small, twisting vessels called sinusoids, the liver lobule, shown opposite, is drenched with blood. Once the lobules have worked their subtle alchemy, blood drains down their central veins into the venous system. Liver cells, above, studded with nuclei, lie amidst meandering sinusoids.

but also in the stomach and even the mouth. Minerals occur in the body in the form of ions. Whether consumed as food or produced by metabolism, ions are vital elements in homeostasis. Because ions mark the difference between extracellular and intracellular fluid, the total amount and individual shares must be kept constant. By keeping what is needed and discarding what is not, the kidneys hold these delicate balances.

Refining the River

Each kidney contains more than a million intricate yet efficient filters, the nephrons. Under high pressure, blood reaches the kidney through the renal artery. Then, still under considerable force, it empties into the head of the nephron, the glomerulus. The glomerulus is a tight knot of capillaries enclosed in a goblet known as Bowman's capsule. The stem of the goblet, or tubule, runs deep into the kidney, rounds a hairpin bend called the loop of Henle, then returns finally to empty into a collecting duct. Capillaries wreathe the tubules like ivy on drainpipes. The collecting duct plunges back into the center of the kidney where it joins the ureter, a muscular tube draining into the bladder. If stretched, the blood vessels and tubules of the kidneys together would extend about 140 miles. Each day, nearly 500 gallons of blood flow through these two masterpieces of a plumber's art.

Blood, after emptying into the glomeruli, filters first into Bowman's capsule where a fifth of the plasma drips into the tubules. Once in the tubules, two processes occur. First, substances required by the body are reabsorbed, passing from the tubules to the capillaries wound around them, while unwanted substances clear the tubule, enter the collecting duct and join the urine. Second, other unwanted substances, generally in small quantities, pass from the capillaries into the walls of the tubules. They are then secreted into the tubule itself to make up part of the urine. Both reabsorption and secretion take place by diffusion and active transport.

The composition of urine, more than its formation, distinguishes the role of the kidneys. After a drinking bout, the body has more water than it can handle. At another time, the body may need

71

to husband all the water it can. A person can pass more than six gallons or less than a pint of urine a day. But always, waste products must be removed in equal proportion in order to maintain the stability of the body fluids. To rid the body of excess water, the kidneys reabsorb more of the substances dissolved in it, forming dilute urine. To keep water but expel wastes, the kidneys make use of a substance called the antidiuretic hormone, which causes most of the water to be reabsorbed while leaving wastes to pass into a concentrated urine. By reabsorbing either solutes or water, the kidneys ensure the stability of the internal environment.

Apart from controlling the balance of body fluids generally, the kidneys also help maintain the body's acid-base balance. They reabsorb or secrete either bicarbonate or hydrogen ions, whichever are needed, to keep pH constant. Even though they are the most powerful of all buffers, the kidneys can take several hours or even days to restore pH to normal.

Far from simply expelling waste, the kidneys recycle the plasma, about sixty times a day, conserving 99 percent of what passes into Bowman's capsule. Except for urea, the waste produced by the liver, all substances reaching the kidneys undergo filtration and reabsorption. More than any other organ, the kidneys determine the composition of blood and, in turn, the balance of the internal environment.

Kidney disorder threatens the internal environment like little else. Kidney disease takes many forms, all of which hinder the kidneys' ability to filter and cleanse the blood. Tainted with wastes, blood fouls the internal environment and hampers the work of organs. Kidney disease shows itself in a variety of symptoms. Urination may be very painful and unusually frequent. Facial and abdominal swelling, back pain, headaches and constant fatigue may also occur. Whatever its origins, kidney failure is called uremia, literally "urine in the blood." Some thirteen million Americans suffer kidney disease and 78,000 die from it each year.

Despite the complexities of its functions, the kidney was the first organ for which man devised a mechanical substitute. The artificial kidney works by dialysis, the process in which blood is taken from the patient and passed through an artificial kidney to remove wastes. Drawn from an artery, blood flows through the artificial kidney, then back into a vein. All artificial kidneys operate on similar principles. They consist of cellophane sheets immersed in a balanced salt solution, the dialyzing fluid. The cellophane sheets are permeable, allowing everything but the plasma proteins to pass between the blood stream and the dialyzing fluid. The fluid is mixed so that excess waste products, like urea, can be removed from the blood, and deficient substances, like bicarbonate ions, can be added.

A recent development, continuous ambulatory peritoneal dialysis (CAPD), promises to make dialysis more convenient and less time-consuming for many patients. CAPD uses the peritoneum, the membrane lining the abdominal cavity, in place of cellophane sheets as the dialyzing membrane. A catheter is placed in the patient's peritoneal cavity and connected to a supply of dialyzing fluid. Gravity feeds the solution into the abdominal cavity from its plastic container. When the process is complete, the dialyzing fluid is returned from the abdominal cavity to the plastic container, then discarded. Although CAPD is not suited to all patients, it will enable many to undergo treatment in much greater freedom. Dialysis, by keeping the body's natural balance through human artifice, reflects the essence of medicine — the art of healing.

By healing the blood, dialysis restores the bond between the body's internal environment and the world surrounding it, the bond on which life itself hangs. The body is akin to an orchestra, its organs so many instruments, each with its own place in the ensemble. Blood, the conductor, cues them to play as one, each sounding its distinct voice in time and in tune with the other. In the body, as in music, balance and harmony count for everything, whether the theme be heroic or pastoral, the tempo brisk or languid. But when the baton is bent or broken, as Shakespeare mused in *Richard II*:

How sour sweet music is
When time is broke and no proportion kept!
So is it in the music of men's lives.

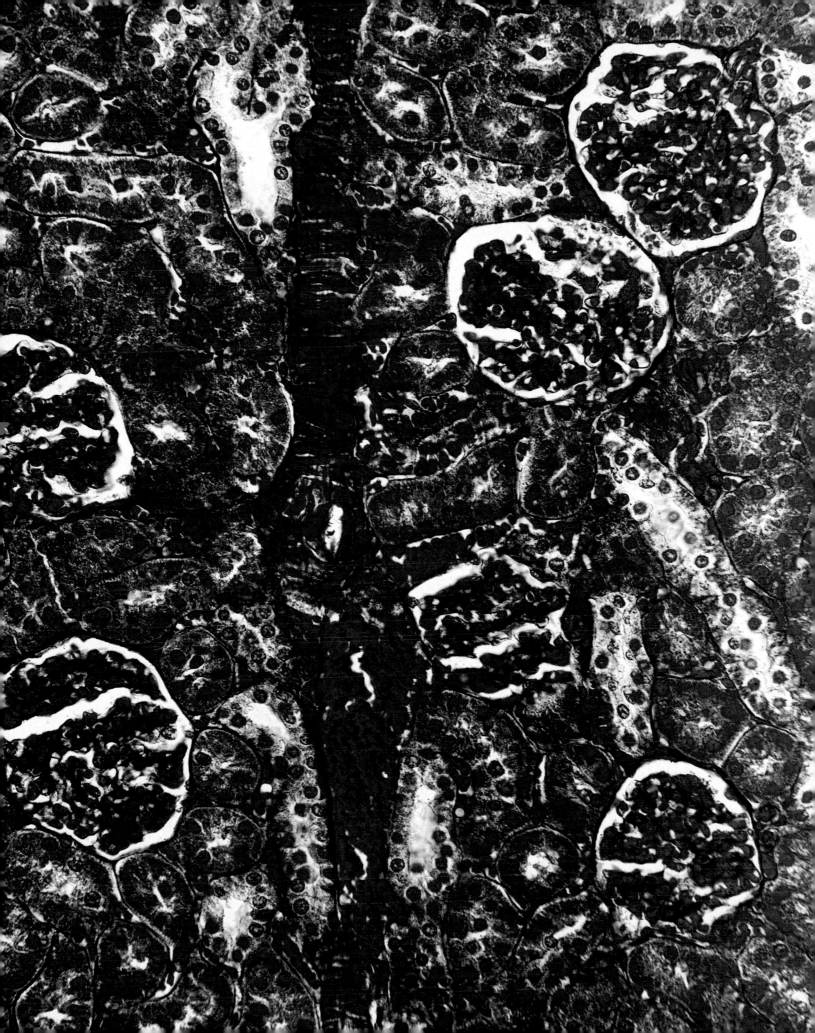

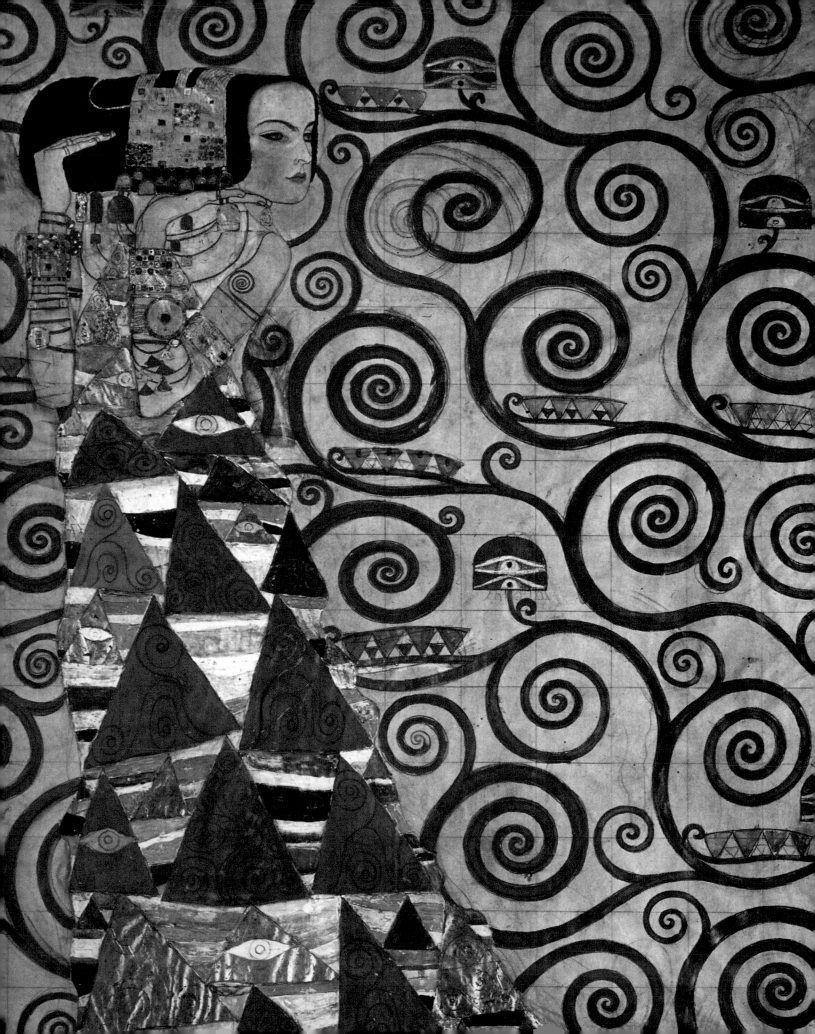

Chapter 4

A Self-Healing Fabric

"The brain may devise laws for the blood, but a hot temper leaps over a cold decree," wrote William Shakespeare in *The Merchant of Venice.* The blood still leaps according to its own temper, but after centuries of research, science has penetrated some of the basic laws that make the liquid a mending fabric of the body. Unlike any fabric yet devised by man, blood will seal rent tissue, magically making its own threads to weave the tear together again. As if guided by invisible hands tooling invisible needles, fine fibers weave themselves into being at the site of the injury, sealing off the escaping blood. When its work is done, the fabric, like a magician's cloak, is lifted to reveal its efficient handiwork. Blood is a self-sustaining liquid, one that requires little attention and works relentlessly throughout life to mend countless seams. The cloth is woven in a complicated process scientists are just beginning to fully understand.

The vital fabric is balanced itself by other processes, all primed to respond to an emergency that threatens the body. When a blood vessel is cut, bruised or otherwise injured, three mutually reinforcing processes move into action. The damaged blood vessel immediately contracts to restrict the flow of blood.

Nervous reflexes triggered by pain impulses spread the contraction to surrounding tissue. The greater the damage the greater the spasm. When cleanly cut, blood vessels suffer less damage and therefore bleed more profusely than ones which have been crushed. Intense vascular spasms can sometimes prevent fatal blood loss from a major artery that has been crushed. Vascular contractions rarely stop bleeding, however, nor do they occur in all vessels. They play no role in slowing blood loss from capillaries because these minuscule vessels have no muscular tissue. Spasms, lasting twenty to thirty minutes, slow blood loss long enough for the body to initiate repairs.

Like a patchwork dress, blood's cloth must be continually mended under the strain of life's wear and tear. Armies of proteins, enzymes and other precisely designed chemicals rally to wounded tissues, where they reweave the delicate fabric.

Minute plugs for leaky vessels, platelets glide through the blood stream in the billions. Temporarily sealing tears in vessel walls, they also release serotonin, a chemical that slows bleeding.

Slender cables of collagen toughen blood vessels, adding strength and elasticity. When a vessel is torn, platelets cling to exposed collagen. They then release a chemical that draws other platelets to the wound.

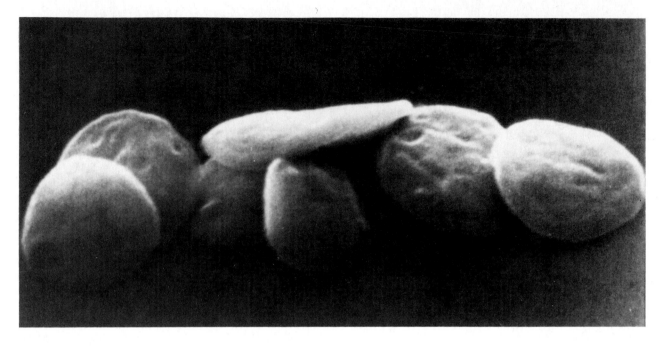

The second process in the repair of an injured blood vessel is the formation of a platelet plug, which lays the foundation for a clot. Platelets are the smallest of the blood cells. They measure only seventy-eight one-hundred-thousandths of an inch in diameter, about one-fourth the size of red blood cells. When magnified fifteen hundred times by a light microscope, the platelet looks like a colorless, grainy speck. Under a scanning electron microscope its form takes shape. At a magnification of eight thousand, the platelet appears as a slightly oval disk. It eluded discovery until the mid-1800s, two centuries after red blood cells were first identified. Even so, the platelet confounded scientists for another half-century.

Resealing Rents

In 1842, British physician William Addison glimpsed through his lens "a great number of extremely minute molecules or granules, varying in size, the largest being at least eight or ten times less than [white blood cells] and . . . in much greater abundance." Forty years later, an Italian pathologist, Giulio Cesare Bizzozero, described the action of these tiny granules. Using preparations from living animals, he watched as platelets rushed to the point of injury and clumped to-

gether to plug the break. Some of these platelets soon broke off and flowed away, while new clumps formed. "During a quarter of an hour one can see this game repeated three or four times," he marveled, "and this can last for hours until the circulation ceases." His description was an accurate one.

Bizzozero also observed that clotting occurred only after platelets sealed the break. He concluded that the platelet was a distinct element in blood, but some of his colleagues refused to accept his theory. Many argued that platelets were merely fragments of white blood cells. Others claimed they were a young form of red blood cells, a belief that persisted until the early twentieth century. At a symposium held at Johns Hopkins University in 1905, one scientist, whose laboratory was on Pikes Peak, Colorado, claimed that platelets contained hemoglobin (the protein that makes red blood cells "red") at high altitudes. Hearing this, Sir William Osler, physician in chief of the university's hospital, replied that he had seen many platelets in his time but none that blushed.

A year later, pathologist James Homer Wright proved conclusively that platelets constituted a third type of blood element because their struc-

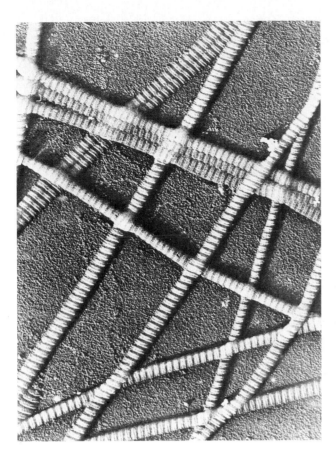

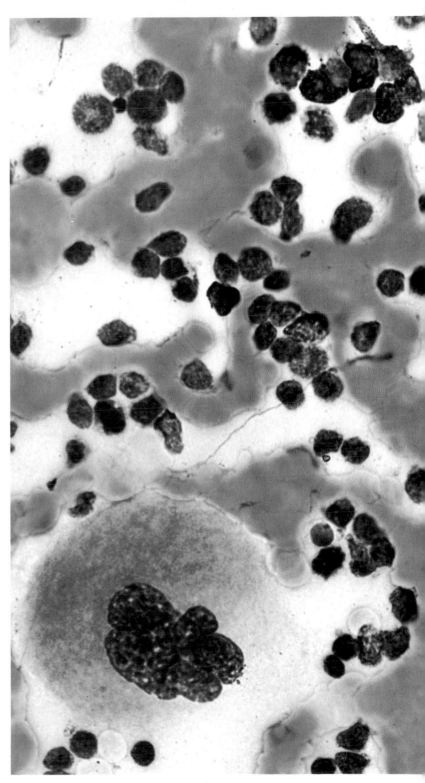

Platelet ancestors, megakaryocytes arise in bone marrow. Each will fragment into many platelets, which flood the blood stream. More than a trillion platelets course through the blood of an average adult.

ture was distinct, and, like red blood cells, they were made in bone marrow. He perfected a stain for blood cells, applied it to marrow and discovered that the platelets' origin could be traced to huge cells in marrow known as megakaryocytes. These giant cells actually fragmented into thousands of platelets.

The average adult possesses more than a trillion platelets, which are produced at a rate of 200 billion a day. Because they are fragments of larger cells, platelets lack nuclei and therefore cannot reproduce. Released into the blood, they age over the course of a week and die after about ten days. During this time, they store substances that will be needed if called into action. Hematologist Theodore Spaet of the Albert Einstein College of Medicine likens the platelet to a sponge "loaded with diverse and biologically active compounds, some of which it can soak up during its voyage through the circulation and all of which it can discharge where . . . needed."

One such compound is serotonin, a substance that causes blood vessels to contract. When it is added to blood plasma, the platelets store almost all of it. Arriving at the site of an injury, platelets release the serotonin, which helps constrict the vessel and reduce bleeding.

Couched in a bed of muscle, an injured blood vessel hemorrhages disk-shaped red blood cells. Grainy platelets cling to collagen on the vessel's wall, swell and discharge adenine diphosphate (ADP), which attracts other platelets to the wound. While the platelets plug the rupture, the damaged tissue releases another chemical called thromboplastin. In the blood stream, thromboplastin triggers a cascade of chemical reactions that ultimately convert the protein fibrinogen to fibrin, whose threads bind the wound. Proteins secreted by the platelets cause the clot to contract, squeezing out fluid and creating a firm seal.

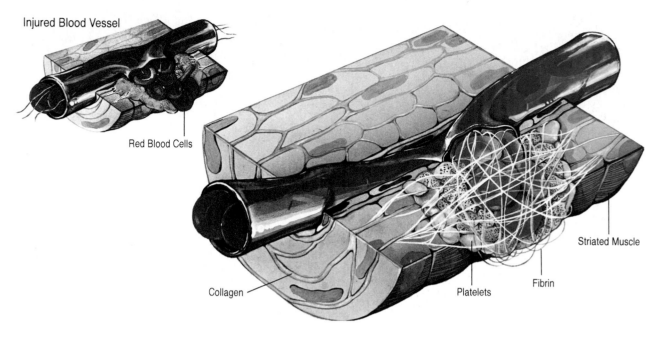

Injured Blood Vessel

Red Blood Cells

Collagen

Platelets

Fibrin

Striated Muscle

Platelets flow freely in the blood stream. They glide along the flat, smooth endothelial cells that form the vessel's inner lining. To ensure their flow, blood vessels produce a prostaglandin known as PGI-2. This substance, a derivative of fatty acids, works aggressively to keep platelets from lumping together.

A rupture in the vessel lining exposes platelets to collagen, a fibrous protein found in connective tissue. Nearby platelets stick to the collagen, swell and secrete adenine diphosphate (ADP), which, together with other chemicals, attracts other platelets. In less than a minute, the platelets build a loose plug that blocks the wound. As a clotting mechanism, the plug is only temporary, but it serves an extremely important function. Hundreds of minuscule breaks occur in the walls of small blood vessels each day. Platelets seal these rents without disrupting the flow of blood. Radiation or drug treatment suppresses the production of platelets, causing small hemorrhages under the skin and in the internal tissues.

If the plug cannot seal a break in the vessel wall, the third process — clotting — will begin. The formation of a clot is a complicated task, one that involves several dozen substances and an intricate sequence of chemical reactions.

Clotting can be triggered by two essentially different mechanisms. Scientists have named these two systems the extrinsic and the intrinsic clotting pathways. The extrinsic pathway is a rapid clotting system activated by the injured vessel wall, which releases a substance called tissue factor, or thromboplastin. Tissue factor then combines with certain clotting factors in the blood to produce another substance called prothrombin activator. At this point, the extrinsic pathway converges with the intrinsic system and both activate a third mechanism that produces the clot.

The intrinsic pathway uses substances only found in the blood. Called clotting factors, they are proteins that constantly circulate in the blood. Until triggered, they remain inactive forms of enzymes, or zymogens, chemicals that speed up reactions without being consumed in the process. Exposure to the injured vessel wall converts one of these zymogens, clotting factor XII, into an enzyme. The conversion then triggers a series of rapid-fire chemical reactions called by some scientists the "cascade effect." Each zymogen, beginning with factor XII, activates the next in the sequence until, finally, the prothrombin activator is produced.

After producing the prothrombin activator, both the extrinsic and intrinsic pathways travel a common route to achieve their final goal — a blood clot. The actual process by which blood transforms from liquid tissue to a solid gel takes place in three steps. The prothrombin activator converts prothrombin, a protein circulating in the blood stream, into thrombin, an enzyme. The thrombin, in turn, transforms fibrinogen, a soluble protein in blood plasma, into insoluble fibrin threads which form the clot.

Researchers have discovered that the thrombin converts fibrinogen into fibrin by severing two short amino-acid chains called peptides from each fibrinogen molecule. Without the peptides, the fibrinogen molecule becomes a fibrin monomer, which means that it is a simple molecule that can combine with other molecules to form a larger structure. The process through which monomers combine is called polymerization. Chemically united by this process, the fibrin monomers stretch out, link up and form long, thin fibrin threads within seconds. These threads wind around the platelet plug in the damaged area of the blood vessel and provide the framework for the clot. At this point, the fibrin threads form a very weak mesh.

To strengthen the fibrin net, platelets and blood proteins called plasma globulins release a fibrin-stabilizing factor. Under the influence of thrombin, this substance links adjacent fibrin threads into a crisscrossed pattern that serves as a more durable framework. Fibrin threads adhere to the injured vessel wall and snare passing blood cells, platelets and plasma to build the clot.

Although firm, somewhat like thick jelly, a blood clot is 99 percent water. Within minutes of formation, the clot begins to contract, squeezing out the fluid portion of blood. The fluid is called serum; it is plasma relieved of fibrinogen and many clotting factors. The energy for contraction comes from platelets, which contain more of the contractile proteins — actin and myosin — than any other tissue except muscle.

Most serum is expelled from the clot within an hour. The mass of fibrin, platelets and the blood substances they entrap is called the hemostatic plug, signifying that it has stanched the flow of

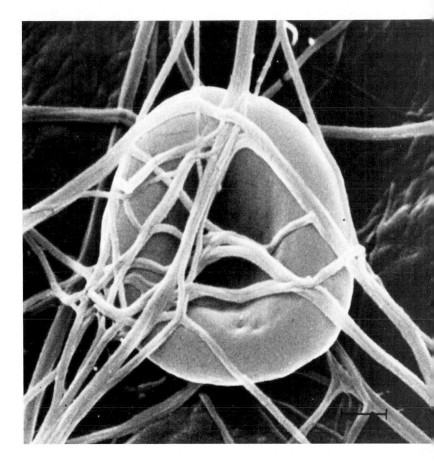

Tendrils of fibrin, the backbone of clots, enmesh a red blood cell. When platelets cannot seal a torn blood vessel, rapid-fire chemical reactions convert the fibrinogen to fibrin, a protein whose threads cling to damaged tissue. Trapped in this tangled net are red blood cells, which strengthen the clot, as gravel strengthens cement. Within minutes, the clot contracts, squeezing out fluid and binding the wound until new tissue can be built.

William Hewson

Fibers in Blood's Fabric

When William Hewson died at age thirty-five from an infection he had contracted during a dissection, Benjamin Franklin, then serving as the American colonial representative to the British government in London, noted in a letter, "He was an excellent young man, ingenious, industrious, useful and beloved." In his concern over the plight of his young friend's family, Franklin added, "All their schemes of life are now overthrown."

Whatever the fallen hopes of his family may have been, Hewson's ambition to win scientific recognition was realized despite his early death. The son of a surgeon from Northumberland, he traveled to London in 1759 at the age of twenty-five to study anatomy. In just three years, he entered a partnership with his teacher and began to lecture on anatomy.

Hewson's first important scientific discovery came in 1768, when he found that birds, fish and reptiles had lymph vessels. For this work he won election to the Royal Society of London, partly through the recommendation of Franklin, himself a member because of his experiments on electricity.

Hewson later extended his investigations to the human

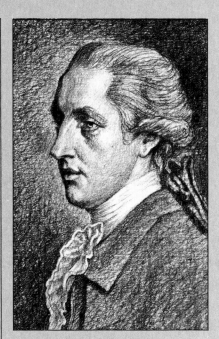

lymphatic system. Using techniques of dye injection and dissection, he proved that lymph vessels were not simply extensions of the arteries, as was commonly supposed, but that they existed separately. Anticipating modern treatments for breast cancer, he recommended that lymph glands be removed as well as the infected breast during surgery, "for otherwise the cancerous humor left in the glands may renew the disease." Examining red blood cells, Hewson again went against contemporary thinking by describing them as "flat as a guinea" rather than globular

in shape, as was thought.

Hewson's greatest contribution to hematology, however, was his research on blood clotting. The prevailing view, stemming from ideas first espoused by Plato, was that blood coagulated after being exposed to cold air outside the body. To disprove this theory, Hewson killed a rabbit and cut out a portion of its jugular vein, tying the ends of a section filled with blood. After freezing the vein in snow, he then thawed and opened it. Draining the blood into a teacup, he observed that it was "perfectly fluid, and in a few minutes it jellied or coagulated as blood usually does." He concluded that changes in the temperature of blood did not cause coagulation.

Hewson noted that cooling delayed coagulation, and that adding salts to the blood slowed the process even further. Using these techniques to arrest the clotting of freshly drawn blood, Hewson allowed the red blood cells to sink in a basin, leaving plasma on top. Skimming the surface of the plasma, he found a substance he named "coagulable lymph," known today as fibrinogen. Hewson was the first to understand that fibrinogen was the natural agent in the blood responsible for clotting.

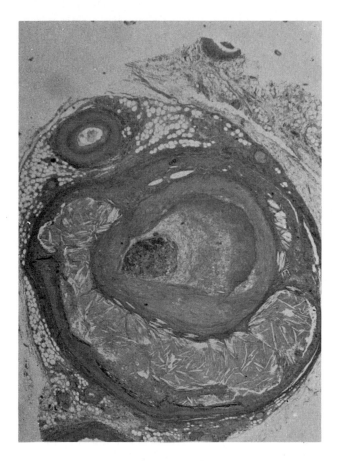

blood. If exposed to air, the clot becomes a coarse, hard lump, brittle to the touch. The clot's appearance to the naked eye belies its hidden structure. In 1914, physiologist W. H. Howell of Johns Hopkins University was the first to see a clot's "meshwork of beautiful needles" through a microscope with ultraviolet light.

Clots, however, are not enough to stop massive blood loss. An individual who loses more than 10 percent of his blood will suffer a sudden drop in blood pressure and usually go into shock. The decreased pressure triggers the body's last measure to stop escaping blood — a powerful wave of nervous reflexes initiated by the sympathetic nervous system. Part of the autonomic nervous system, the sympathetic reflexes constrict veins and arterioles throughout the body to slow the drop in blood pressure. Heart rate soars as high as 200 beats a minute to maintain blood flow, especially to the brain and heart itself. When the sympathetic reflexes work properly, a person can lose as much as 40 percent of his total blood volume and still live. Without this reflex, the loss of 15 to 20 percent of blood volume would be fatal.

By necessity, coagulation must be temporary. Whether triggered by injury or disease, the clot must gradually dissolve and disappear as cells make new tissue and the wound heals. Yet, once started, clotting is a relentless process. Within minutes, coagulation spreads into the surrounding blood stream. In a vicious cycle, prothrombin splits into thrombin, which causes the further activation of prothrombin, and the prothrombin produces still more thrombin. Newly formed thrombin also energizes clotting factors involved in the production of the prothrombin activator. Normally the flow of blood checks the process by carrying the clotting factors away rapidly.

If blood flow is abnormally slow, however, an unnecessary blood clot can form. Such a clot is called a thrombus, from the Greek *thrombos*, meaning "lump." Thrombi usually adhere to blood vessel walls. If they continue to grow they can reduce blood flow through the vessel. A blood clot can also break free from the vessel wall, lodge in a smaller vessel and block the flow of blood. This is an embolism. A clot that blocks the opening into the pulmonary arteries, which deliver used blood to the lungs, can be fatal. Clots that lodge in the coronary arteries can cut off blood to the heart and cause a myocardial infarction, commonly called a heart attack. If a blood clot reaches the brain, it might block a vessel and result in stroke. Blood clots are not always caused by external injuries. Bacteria or bacterial toxins can activate the clotting process over a wide area, producing many clots along small vessels. Victims sometimes experience serious bleeding because the bacterially induced clots deplete the supply of clotting factors.

Some scientists believe that clots continually build up and dissolve in the blood. Other hematologists think that if this were true, then clotting factors would be longer-lived in those people who have clotting defects. But they say this does not happen. Researchers have discovered that intravascular clotting frequently occurs when the blood is in a state of hypercoagulability, meaning that high levels of coagulants are circulating in the blood stream. A number of conditions promote hypercoagulability. When a person remains stationary for long periods of time, blood flow slows down. Sluggish blood flow might allow clotting factors to accumulate in one place and so trigger clotting. Physicians usually insist that bed patients be moved frequently to increase their circulation. Other causes of hypercoagulability include congestive heart failure, birth control pills containing the hormone estrogen, pregnancy (which often raises the levels of coagulation factors), cancer and certain drugs.

Generally, however, hypercoagulability alone will not trigger the formation of a thrombus. A tiny lesion — so small that it is only visible through an electron microscope — will attract platelets that stick to the vessel walls and trigger clotting. In veins, an inflammation of the vascular wall initiating the formation of a thrombus is called phlebitis. Atherosclerosis, localized lesions that thicken and roughen the inner lining of arteries, may also spur the formation of clots. So many conditions seem to stimulate clotting that one scientist questions "not so much why clotting occurs . . . but why it does not occur constantly, with devastating effects."

To Clot or Not to Clot

The clotting mechanisms must start at a moment's notice, yet the blood must never permit the process to run wild. In this state of tension, it maintains ready supplies of coagulants that are counterbalanced by anticoagulant substances and processes. Our blood is indeed "a very special juice," as the devil in Goethe's *Faust* observes. But the blood's remarkable balancing act does not stop there. Anticoagulation must also be controlled. Unchecked, it will cause hemorrhaging. Anticoagulation begins with the clotting process itself. Clotting factors, such as thrombin, are not self-perpetuating until and unless they reach a certain level of concentration. To prevent this concentration from being reached, a substance known as antithrombin circulates in the blood stream. Antithrombin attaches itself to thrombin, molecule to molecule, thus preventing the thrombin from converting fibrinogen into fibrin.

One of the most powerful inhibitors of clotting is heparin, a large carbohydrate produced by mast cells, special cells found in the intestines and the lungs but also made by these cells elsewhere in the body. Researchers have not yet identified the physiological mechanism for heparin action. They do know that heparin prevents blood from clotting by combining with another chemical called a cofactor. The cofactor that heparin binds with is the antithrombin-heparin cofactor. By itself, the cofactor binds with thrombin to remove excess amounts of thrombin from the circulation in ten to twenty minutes. It is possible that small amounts of heparin circulate in the blood stream. If needed, more heparin could be released into the blood. Excess heparin speeds up the reaction a thousand times, eliminating thrombin almost instantly.

Heparin and other anticoagulants can prevent blood from clotting, but they cannot destroy a clot that already exists. The seeds of a clot's destruction are hidden in its fibrin. Breaking fibrin down, much like building it up, takes place in steps that together complete a process known as fibrinolysis. A clot contains plasminogen, a blood protein that lies in wait to be activated by enzymes called plasminogen activators.

Plasminogen activators are the key to fibrinolysis. They convert the protein plasminogen into an enzyme, plasmin. Plasmin is very selective and extremely effective. It digests fibrin by making it soluble and reducing it to fragments. The fragments escaping from a clot are removed from the blood by the liver. Fibrinolysis can be a relatively slow process. It might take weeks or even months to make old clots soluble.

Like other clotting and anticlotting processes, fibrinolysis must be perfectly balanced. Premature activity can dissolve clots before a wound has healed. To keep fibrinolysis in check, the liver produces a substance called antiplasmin that neutralizes excess plasmin in the blood stream.

No longer useful, the fibrin fragments must be removed from the blood stream. To accomplish this, white blood cells called phagocytes devour the scattering debris. These cells can remain in one place or they can seek their prey, stalking the tissues and the blood itself. Phagocytic white

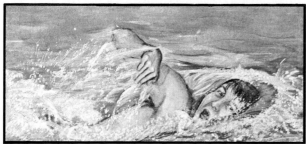

Exercise boosts the production of chemical activators that destroy unwanted clots.

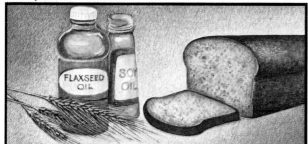

Lecithin-rich foods make platelets less sticky, lowering the risk that clots will trigger heart disease.

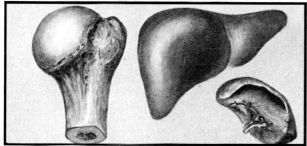

Bone marrow, the liver and the spleen continually filter small clots from the blood stream.

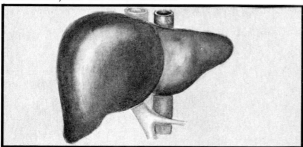

Liver cells balance clotting forces with antiplasmin, which neutralizes the clotting agent plasmin.

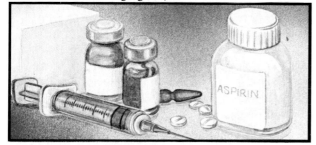

A pharmacopoeia of anticoagulant drugs, including aspirin, disrupt the blood's clotting machinery.

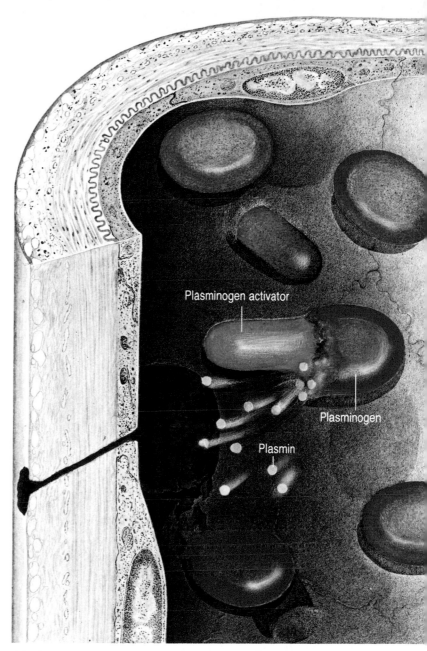

Blood must scrap clots once they have helped mend damaged tissue. A family of enzymes called plasminogen activators fires reactions that convert plasminogen to plasmin, which devours fibrin threads. The debris is swept away by blood. Among the plasminogen activators is urokinase. Researchers have found abnormal amounts of urokinase in tumors, suggesting that cancer cells fight the body's efforts to encircle tumors with clots.

cells can remove small clots from the blood stream. With macrophages, other giant white cells, they collectively make up the tissue macrophage system. The liver continually removes active coagulants from the circulation, bypassing reserves of their inactive forms. When the liver is diseased, as in the case of cirrhosis, the level of active coagulants decreases, and cuts that should clot rapidly can ooze for a relatively long time. Experiments on laboratory animals have demonstrated just how potent the macrophage system is. With this system blocked, many of the animals rapidly suffer massive, fatal thrombi when they are injected with activated clotting factors.

Fuel for Balance

Studies have also revealed that anticlotting mechanisms can be affected by changes in diet. During World War II, drastic food rationing was common throughout Scandinavia. The worst food shortage occurred in Norway. Nazi occupiers stripped the country of livestock and prohibited the milling of white flour. For four years, whole wheat bread was the major staple of the Norwegian diet until the Allied victory in 1945.

During the occupation, Paul Owren, a hematologist in Oslo, noticed a significant drop in deaths from vascular disease. Reporting on his findings twenty years later, Owren noted that, in 1941, clotting had caused twenty-six out of one thousand deaths in Oslo City Hospital. By 1944, the number of deaths had dropped to seven per thousand. Owren traced the decline in mortality rates to changes in the Norwegian diet.

Analysis of the ingredients in whole wheat bread confirmed Owren's hunch. Other researchers discovered that whole wheat bread contains lecithin, an agent that minimizes friction. Sprayed onto a frying pan, lecithin prevents food from sticking to the surface. Since platelets become sticky and clump together at the beginning of the clotting process, scientists wondered if lecithin might affect the platelets. Arvid Hellem, a colleague of Owren's, measured the stickiness of platelets by passing a blood sample through a tube containing glass beads. If 80 percent of the platelets passed through, the 20 percent that adhered to the beads indicated a platelet adhesiveness index (PAI) of twenty. Using this index, scientists learned that the stickiness of a patient's platelets nearly doubled for a two-week period following a major injury. They also discovered that a high degree of platelet adhesiveness constituted one of the major causes of dangerous clots after an injury.

To determine the effect of lecithin on clotting, hematologist James Kirby of the New Jersey State Hospital consumed measured amounts of soybean and flaxseed oils, both containing amounts of lecithin similar to that found in whole wheat bread, for five days. During this time, his PAI dropped from fifty to twenty. When he stopped the high-lecithin diet, his PAI rapidly rose to fifty again. Subsequent studies have also revealed that a shift in lecithin consumption can alter the blood's ability to clot, virtually overnight.

Another dietary factor that affects clotting is vitamin K, found primarily in leafy green vegetables, tomatoes and vegetable oils. Bacteria found in the intestines also manufacture vitamin K; indeed, the intestines are the body's major source. Both a proper diet and effectively functioning bacteria are essential because body tissues store so little of this vitamin. When medical treatment for serious infections sterilizes the gastrointestinal tract, vitamin K deficiency appears within forty-eight hours.

Vitamin K was accidentally discovered in 1935 by Danish biochemist Henrik Dam. When Dam fed chicks a low-fat diet to study how their bodies used cholesterol, he noticed that they became anemic and developed severe bleeding problems. Dam discovered that he could stop the hemorrhaging by feeding the chicks a substance found in grains and seeds. He named the substance the Koagulation-Vitamin. In 1939, American biochemist E. A. Doisy isolated the pure form of vitamin K and determined its structure. For their work, both Dam and Doisy received the 1943 Nobel Prize in medicine. Chemists now know that vitamin K is fat-soluble, which means that it reaches body tissues via fats in the diet. Therefore, a low-fat diet is also a low vitamin K diet.

Vitamin K is necessary for the formation of prothrombin and three other clotting factors pro-

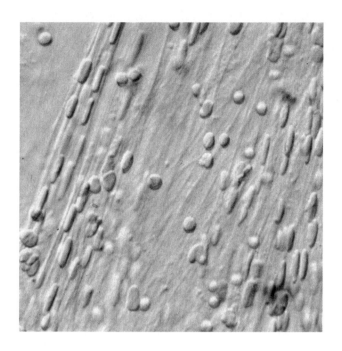 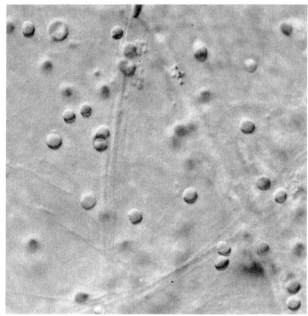

duced by the liver. Without the K-inspired liver actions, proper clotting cannot take place. Liver disease can disrupt the vitamin's operations. For this reason, doctors give injections of the vitamin to all patients suffering from liver disorders before attempting any form of surgery. And breast-fed babies sometimes require a vitamin K supplement because human milk contains less of the vitamin than does cow's milk. Some newborn infants bleed from the severed umbilical cord before their intestinal bacteria have had a chance to develop. But the bleeding usually stops after two or three days, by which time the bacteria have begun to work. Injections of vitamin K are usually necessary, however, until the bacteria appear.

Tricking the System

If needed, drugs can also be used to prevent the blood from clotting. They fall into three main categories. The first group consists of drugs that interfere with the formation of fibrin. Among the most commonly used is heparin. Heparin injections provide a powerful anticoagulant that is used primarily for surgical patients with a high risk of clotting. The artificially high level of heparin has an immediate effect but it will disappear from the body within one to four hours. It is pos-

Snagged by fibrin threads, red blood cells stretch into elongated capsules in a clot. Ten minutes after plasmin, a clot-dissolving enzyme, begins to chew the fibrin, the clot vanishes. Fibrin fragments are washed away and filtered from blood by the liver, which also manufactures a substance called antiplasmin that holds clot removal forces in check.

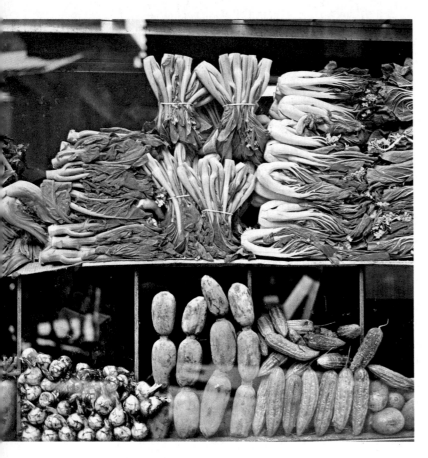

A Chinatown window display in New York beckons passersby with enticing, nutrition-laden vegetables. Leafy green vegetables, tomatoes and vegetable oils are nature's best sources of vitamin K, essential to the liver's manufacture of clotting agents. Intestinal bacteria also supply vitamin K, but dietary sources are needed because tissues store little of the nutrient.

sible that a blood enzyme rapidly destroys the drug and that much of the administered heparin gets trapped in the liver and cannot make its way through the blood stream. Because heparin cannot be administered orally, another drug is necessary for long-term treatment.

In 1921, a mysterious bleeding disease swept through herds of cattle in Alberta, Canada. At first, doctors suspected that bacteria entering their blood stream were causing the hemorrhaging. But no organism could be found. The cattle continued to die until a veterinarian noticed that they became ill after eating spoiled sweet clover. He linked the curious bleeding to impaired blood-clotting mechanisms. Another scientist traced the cause to a deficiency of prothrombin.

The substance that caused the hemorrhaging was not identified until another outbreak of the bleeding disease hit the Midwest in the 1930s. The Depression had forced many farmers to use spoiled sweet clover as feed. One farmer, afraid the disease would destroy his entire herd, loaded a dead cow, a can of its blood and some clover onto a truck and drove almost 200 miles to the University of Wisconsin to find help. At the university's agricultural experiment station, biochemist Karl Paul Link examined the hay. The rotting process, Link discovered, had changed coumarin, a harmless substance that gives clover its characteristic odor and taste, into a toxic substance. By the late 1930s, scientists isolated the toxic agent, found that it acted as a long-term anticoagulant and named it dicumarol.

Dicumarol, when added to blood in a test tube, produces no reaction. But in cattle and humans, it blocks the action of vitamin K in the liver's cells. Without vitamin K, the liver cannot produce prothrombin and other clotting factors. Reducing the production of prothrombin and the other clotting factors dependent on vitamin K to 10 percent of their normal level is apparently sufficient to stop fibrin formation. The action of dicumarol is delayed, usually four to five days, until the body uses the vitamin K-dependent factors already in the blood stream. Dicumarol complements the immediate action of heparin, so drug therapy must overlap a few days to fully protect the body against thrombi.

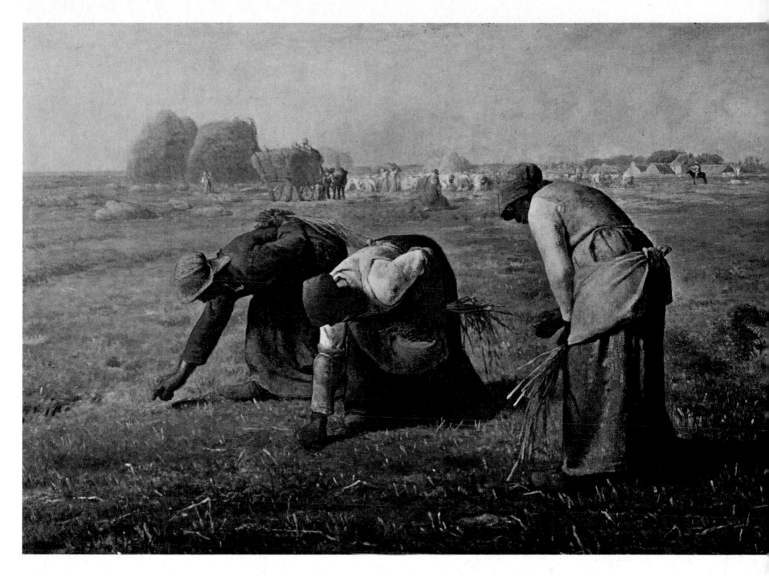

The second group of anticoagulant drugs works by preventing platelets from sticking together to form a plug. The most commonly used drug is aspirin. Aspirin is effective because it impairs the release of clot-promoting substances from the platelet.

Drugs that digest the fibrin threads forming the framework of the clot constitute the third type of anticoagulant. In the 1950s, researchers isolated urokinase, an enzyme that helps clear the urinary tract, from human urine. Urokinase, they discovered, is a plasminogen activator that can accelerate fibrinolysis. It is now used clinically to combat arterial and venous thrombi, particularly lung clots. Urokinase is also derived from cultured kidney cells, a source that yields the enzyme more quickly and cheaply.

Another important fibrinolytic agent is streptokinase, a substance released by streptococcal bacteria. It is used as a plasminogen activator to

Scraps from the reaper's table are gathered by French peasants in Jean Millet's painting, The Gleaners. *However poor their economic condition, the gleaners' diet was enriched by a substance called lecithin, found in whole wheat. Lecithin makes blood platelets less sticky, thus lowering the risk that dangerous clots will form.*

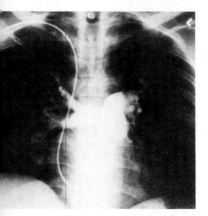
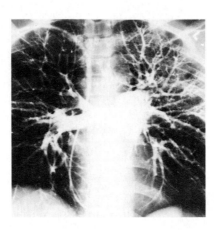

accelerate fibrinolysis and also used to dissolve arterial and venous thrombi. Streptokinase also converts plasminogen into plasmin, the enzyme that destroys fibrin threads in blood clots. When infused via catheters into the coronary arteries of heart attack victims a few hours after their first symptoms, streptokinase has helped dissolve clots. But use of it as a drug still holds problems. Streptokinase, in dissolving clots, might disturb heart rhythms. Streptokinase, more than urokinase, causes the destruction of fibrinogen and other clotting factors that may be needed elsewhere, thus creating the possibility of severe hemorrhaging in patients.

Such bleeding is a danger inherent in all anticoagulation therapy, and it is especially dangerous when the individual receiving the therapy already has a disease or condition — such as peptic ulcers — involving lesions. Anticoagulation drugs pose other, potentially fatal dangers. Their sudden discontinuation may trigger extensive clotting and bring on death. Even under the most carefully supervised conditions, thrombi can occur while a person is still taking the drugs.

A Barbarous Affliction

At the other extreme are the bleeding disorders — a wide group of ailments that prevent the blood from coagulating quickly enough. Bleeding disorders can arise from a variety of causes including liver disease, vitamin K deficiency and the use of certain antibiotics. A small percentage of bleeding disorders are hereditary, making victims deficient in one of the many clotting factors.

The most common bleeding disorder is hemophilia, meaning "love of blood." A nineteenth-century researcher called the term "barbarous and senseless." His sharp words characterize the disease itself. Hemophilia endangers the victim in numerous ways beyond the loss of blood. Blood hemorrhaging in muscles can sap the body's strength and damage nerves. Bleeding in joints can permanently cripple the hemophiliac by weakening and deforming his bones.

Descriptions of hemophilia are found scattered through the centuries. One of the earliest, from the second century A.D., tells of a rabbi who excused a woman's third son from circumcision, for the boy's two brothers had already bled to death following the procedure. Another rabbi, noting that the sons of three sisters had died similarly, would not allow the fourth sister's boy to be circumcised. The Talmud records his words to the child's mother. "Abstain from circumcision," the rabbi warned her, "for there are families whose blood is loose."

Tenth-century Arab physician Abul Kasim wrote a manual of surgery that was used for centuries. Kasim noted in the book the mysterious deaths of men in one village. All of them had bled to death from minor wounds. In 1791, an American newspaper reported a similar phenomenon. A nineteen-year-old Massachusetts youth, Isaac Zoll, cut his foot one day, but the wound never healed, and he bled to death. The Salem *Gazette* noted that Isaac's five brothers had also died from minor cuts. "The father of the above persons has had two wives, and by each, several children," the young man's obituary read. "Those who died in this singular manner were all of the first wife."

The curious affliction remained unidentified until 1803, when Philadelphia physician John Otto published a study tracing the history of several families of "bleeders." In his account, Otto traced its origin to a woman named Smith who had settled in Plymouth, New Hampshire, seventy or eighty years earlier. She had "transmitted the . . . idiosyncrasy to her descendants," wrote the physician. "It is one . . . to which her family is unfortunately subject, and has been the source not only of great solicitude, but frequent-

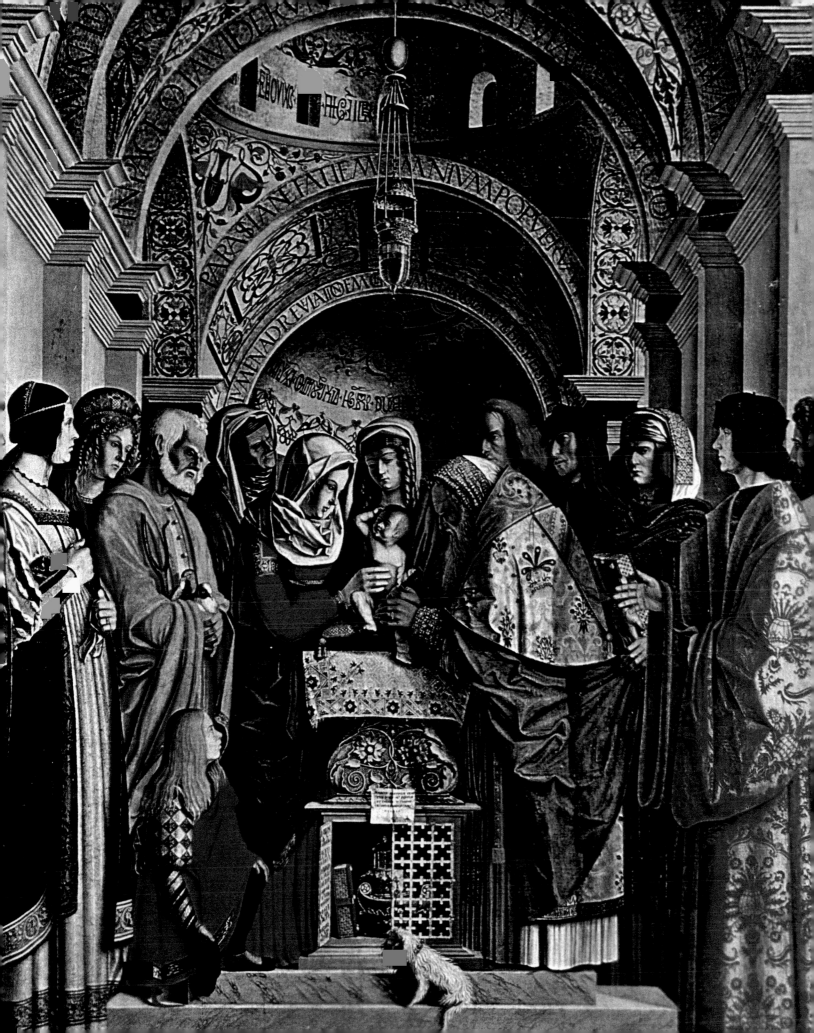

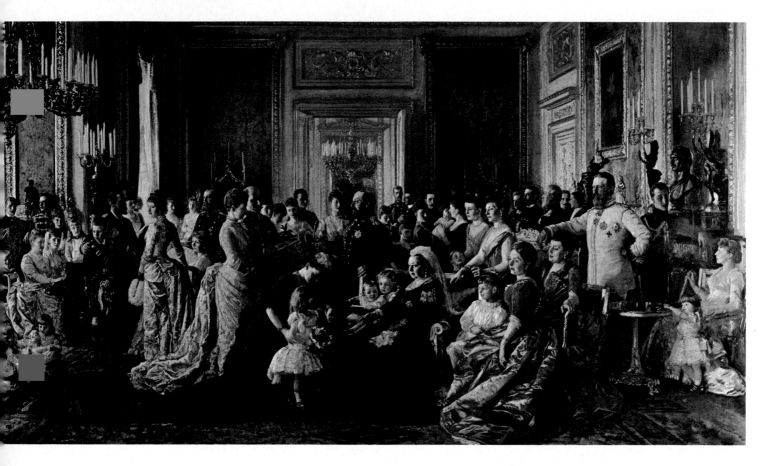

ly the cause of death. If the least scratch is made on the skin of some of them, as mortal a hemorrhage will eventually ensue as if the largest wound is inflicted." He noted the major characteristics of hemophilia, as well as its "surprising circumstance that the males only are subject to this strange affection," yet "all of them are not liable to it." Otto also observed that the disease did not strike the women, but they were "still capable of transmitting it to their male children." Otto recorded the anguish the disease brought to other families. The father of several hemophiliac sons lived with the fear that every day would bring "an accident which will destroy them."

Otto's work fired the imagination of other doctors who traced the disease to its roots in several families in America and Europe. The mechanics that determined inheritance of the disease were not understood, however, until the early 1900s, when the work of Austrian botanist Gregor Mendel finally gained the attention of the scientific community. Mendel had published his studies outlining the principles of heredity nearly half a century earlier.

As the study of genetics matured, scientists recognized that hemophilia was hereditary. Chromosomes, carrying genes, pair up like twin meeting twin. The chromosomes from the mother link with an equal number from the father, each pair determined by the type of information the genes carry. The two genes determining eye color lie at identical places on either side of the chromosome pair. This arrangement is true for all twenty-three pairs, save one. The differing pair determines the sex of the child. Females have two X chromosomes; males have an X and a Y. The mother passes on an X chromosome, and the father, either an X or a Y. Two X chromosomes produce a female, and the combination of an X and a Y make a male.

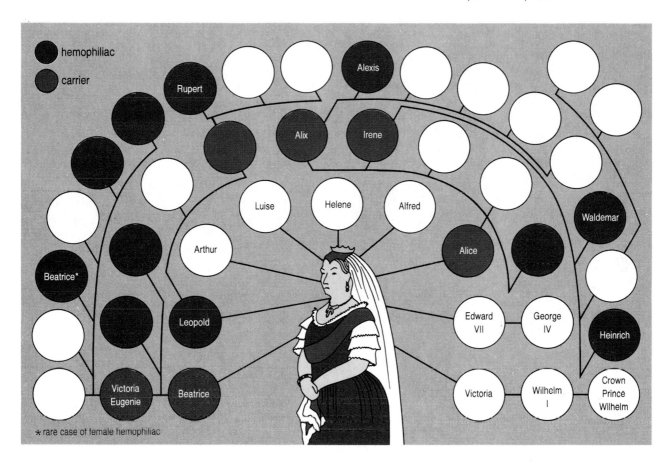

Hemophilia stems from an abnormal gene on the X chromosome. Thus, a female is usually spared the disease because, although she may have received one abnormal X chromosome from her mother, the normal X passed on by her father will have counteracted it. She will, however, be a carrier of the disease and can pass it on to her children. A woman can be a hemophiliac only if her mother is a carrier and her father is a hemophiliac, which is very rare. A male, however, receives only one X chromosome. If his mother is a carrier, the child will have a 50 percent chance of being a hemophiliac.

Hemophilia has gained a somewhat exotic reputation through its long association with several European houses of royalty. In 1837, an eighteen-year-old girl named Victoria became queen of England. A respected and loved ruler, she gave her name to an era. Queen Victoria inadvertently achieved fame of another sort, however, as a carrier of the disease that would afflict royal families across the continent, and shape history as it shaped their lives.

In tracing the disease, scientists think it probably originated from a mutated gene in either the queen or one of her parents. In 1853, Victoria gave birth to her eighth child, Leopold. The boy suffered from severe hemophilia. When Leopold was twenty-six, the queen confided in a letter that he had "been four or five times at death's door" and went "hardly a few months without being laid up." At age thirty-one, Leopold fell, striking his head, and died shortly afterwards of severe hemorrhaging. Two of his sisters, Beatrice and Alice, proved to be carriers of the disease. Both women married German princes and transmitted the defective gene to their children. Two of Beatrice's three sons were hemophiliacs and her daughter, a carrier, gave birth to three hemophiliac sons. One of Alice's sons bled to death at

91

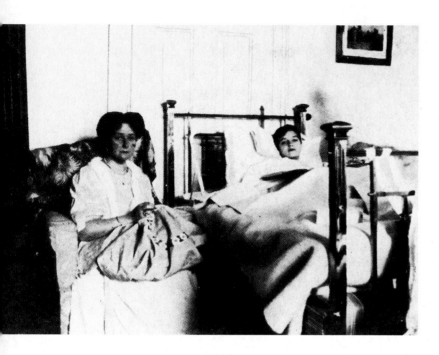

A bumpy carriage ride precipitated a severe attack of hemophilia in young Alexis, heir to the Romanov dynasty, at a Polish hunting lodge in 1912. The czarevich acquired the flawed gene from his mother, the Empress Alexandra, shown at his bedside. A German princess who married Czar Nicholas II in 1894, Alexandra was the granddaughter of Queen Victoria.

the age of three, and two of her daughters passed the disease on to their children.

One of Alice's daughters, Princess Alix, inadvertently transformed the family affliction into a political drama. In 1884, twelve-year-old Alix traveled to St. Petersburg to attend her sister's marriage to the Grand Duke Serge, the brother of Alexander III, Czar of Russia. There, she met Nicholas II, the czar's son and heir. Enchanted with the German princess, Nicholas fell in love almost instantly. He vowed to marry her, much to the disapproval of his family. They tried to turn his attention to other princesses, but he remained steadfast. As Czar Alexander III lay dying in 1894, the family consented to the marriage. A month after his death, the young couple were married. Alix converted to Russian Orthodoxy and took the name Alexandra Feodorovna.

During the first ten years of marriage, the royal couple failed to produce a male heir. In desperation, Alexandra turned to miracle workers. When the miracle came, its glow was brief. In 1904, a son, Alexis, was born. But by the age of six weeks, he was bleeding from the navel. As a toddler, trivial bumps and knocks resulted in large bruises. Alexis was a hemophiliac.

In July 1907, as the three-year-old Alexis lay close to death, a strange man made his way into the royal circle. A ragged Siberian peasant with a long, tangled beard and eyes of steel, he radiated a magnetism that was difficult to fathom. He had been born Gregory Efimovich but, as a young man, received the nickname "Rasputin," meaning "licentious one." The informal name was apparently well earned. He was a self-proclaimed *staretz*, a holy man, who had won acceptance in some of St. Petersburg's most influential circles. One night, Alexandra summoned the staretz to the palace, where he held the ailing czarevich's hand and told Russian folk stories. By morning the boy seemed better. His pain had lessened and he was able to sit up in bed. More significantly, the monk had won the unwavering faith and loyalty of the empress.

Five years later, as Alexis was attempting to jump into a boat, he fell, sharply striking his left thigh. He was still recovering from the hemorrhage when, several weeks later, during a carriage ride he began to bleed again. The pain was unbearable. Every jolt made him scream. Alexandra turned to the only help she knew — the unconventional staretz. She wired him at his home in Siberia, and he replied, "God has seen your tears and heard your prayers. Do not grieve. The Little One will not die. Do not allow the doctors to bother him too much." A day later, the boy seemed much improved.

Others did not look upon Rasputin as a savior. St. Petersburg buzzed with gossip about the monk's seductions and orgies. At a time of internal political turmoil, Rasputin's reputation and influence over the royal family further weakened the hold Nicholas had over the country. The gossip, which made its way to Alexandra, only strengthened her fierce devotion to the man who was "Our Friend." With the outbreak of World War I, Nicholas took command of the army and remained away from home for long periods of time, placing much of the affairs of state in his wife's hands. She turned to the staretz for advice and followed his suggestions blindly. This, too, was openly talked about. "Rasputin's leap from the personal chronicles of the imperial family into the arena of Russian history was one of those historical absurdities," recalled Alexander Kerensky, a leading revolutionary; it was "a case of an intimate family drama moving into the limelight of world politics."

As the unpopularity of Russia's royal family grew, members of the court sought to reverse the adverse course of events by arranging Rasputin's murder. In December 1916, they carried out their plan. They lured him to a St. Petersburg estate where they fed him poisoned cakes and wine. When the poison failed to take effect, one of the men grabbed a pistol and shot Rasputin in the back. The monk collapsed. Thinking they had killed him, the conspirators brought in a doctor to pronounce him dead, which the doctor did. But suddenly, the monk's strange eyes shot open. Seconds later, he was chasing his "murderer" into a snowy courtyard. Horrified, one of the men fired the gun again, hitting Rasputin twice. The men gathered around the body as it lay in bloodied snow. They kicked the peasant's head with their heavy boots and bludgeoned him with

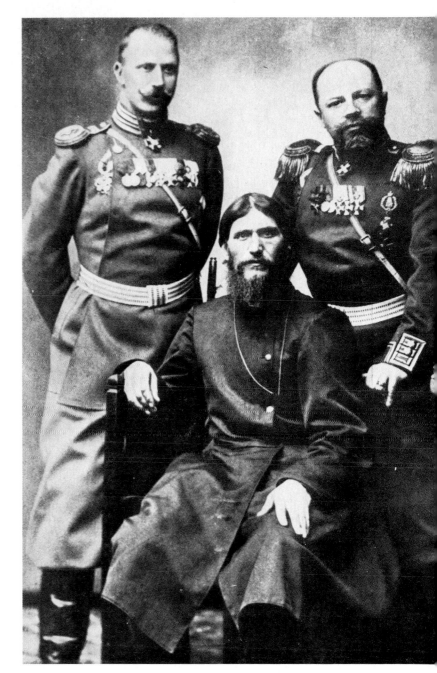

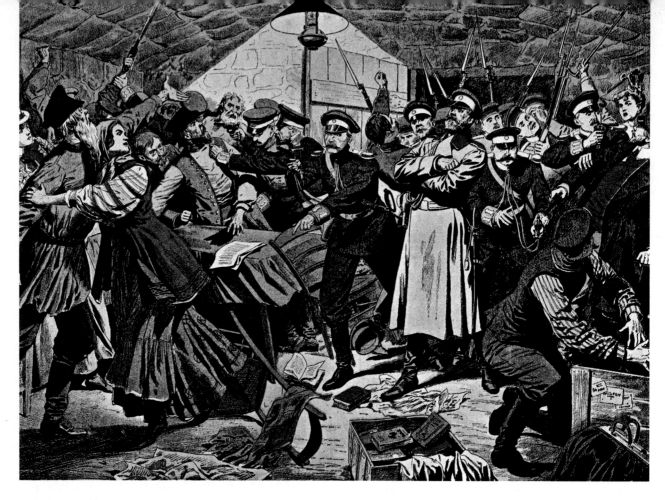

a club. Finally, the conspirators rolled his body in a cloth, bound the bundle with cords and dropped it into an icebound river. When the body was found three days later, investigators discovered the cause of his death. His lungs were filled with water; Rasputin had drowned.

Demonstrations against the czar grew into violent riots. The Russian parliament managed to restore order but insisted that Nicholas abdicate and turn the throne over to his son. At first he agreed, but mindful of his son's delicate health, he named his brother Michael successor, instead. The decision fueled greater discontent. The revolution erupted. In 1917, Bolsheviks seized the royal family. They were sent to the "House of Special Purpose" in the Ural Mountains, a thousand miles from St. Petersburg. Shortly after midnight on July 17, 1918, local Bolsheviks executed the family in the basement of the house. The Romanov dynasty, which had begun in a conspiracy two hundred years earlier, had come to an end. So had the disease that had played its bizarre role in the revolution.

Ironically, at the time Alexis was born, science was making its first strides toward understanding and treating hemophilia. Shortly before the turn of the century, British physician Almroth Wright

measured blood's coagulation time, a procedure that provided major insight into the illness. Wright discovered that hemophiliacs had an abnormally slow clotting time. Earlier researchers had speculated that the defect lay in the blood vessels. Some had even linked it to rheumatism.

Using Wright's insight, scientists focused on the clotting process in an effort to discover the cause of the delay. They found that thrombin, the enzyme that converts fibrinogen into fibrin, formed slowly in hemophiliacs. In 1911, Scottish physician Thomas Addis suggested that the key to hemophilia lay in the faulty conversion of prothrombin to thrombin. Addis also discovered that a solution made from proteins extracted from normal blood plasma could improve a hemophiliac's clotting time. His findings were accepted for twenty years until another scientist showed that prothrombin in hemophiliacs was indeed normal — a find that led to renewed controversy over the disease's cause. Some scientists believed abnormal platelets were responsible. Others thought the problem lay in the plasma.

Finally, in 1936, a group of researchers demonstrated that normal platelets did not shorten the hemophiliac's blood clotting time. Scientists then focused their interest on plasma. In 1937, two

Harvard researchers re-created the plasma fraction Addis had used in his experiments and they confirmed his findings. One of the researchers later named the substance antihemophilic globulin. Today, it is called the antihemophilic factor (AHF) or, more simply, factor VIII.

Although scientists felt assured that hemophilia resulted from an abnormal deficiency of factor VIII, one puzzle remained unsolved. On occasion, a hemophiliac, given another hemophiliac's blood, would show an improved clotting time. In 1952, two scientists independently published papers that explained this paradox. They had found another form of hemophilia, nearly identical to that associated with factor VIII but due to a deficiency of a previously unknown clotting factor, which they named factor IX. This form of hemophilia, called hemophilia B, or Christmas disease (named for an early victim) is more rare than that caused by factor VIII. The factor VIII-deficient disease is hemophilia A, or classic hemophilia. Scientists are uncertain which form plagued the royal families of Europe.

The development of blood transfusions and techniques for separating and storing plasma made modern treatment for hemophilia possible. Prior to these advances in the early twentieth century, people stricken with severe hemophilia rarely survived childhood. There is still no cure for the disease, but the treatment for hemophilia has improved. In the mid-1960s, American physiologist Judith Pool discovered that slowly thawed frozen plasma yielded deposits high in factor VIII. The deposits called cryoprecipitates are further refined to provide excellent emergency therapy and permit hemophiliacs to undergo surgery — even open heart surgery.

In addition to medical treatment, home treatment programs enable hemophiliacs to lead more normal lives. Such programs reduce the expense of treating the disease by thousands of dollars per patient annually. They also reduce the amount of time hemophiliacs must spend away from school or work. Patients are taught to assess degrees of bleeding, to respond to specific symptoms, to calculate correct treatment dosages and to keep records. Long controlled by their affliction, hemophiliacs can now control their lives.

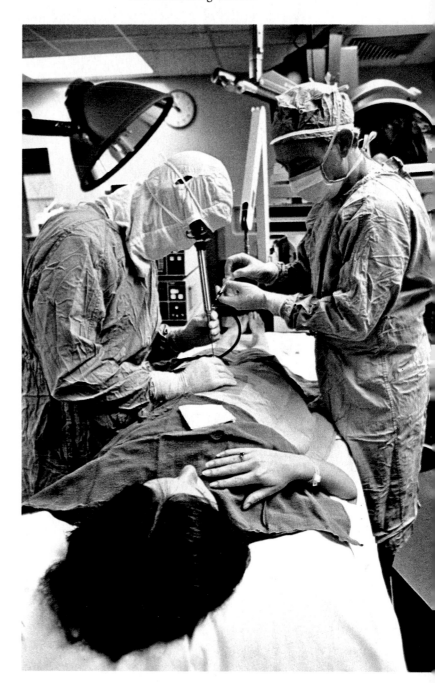

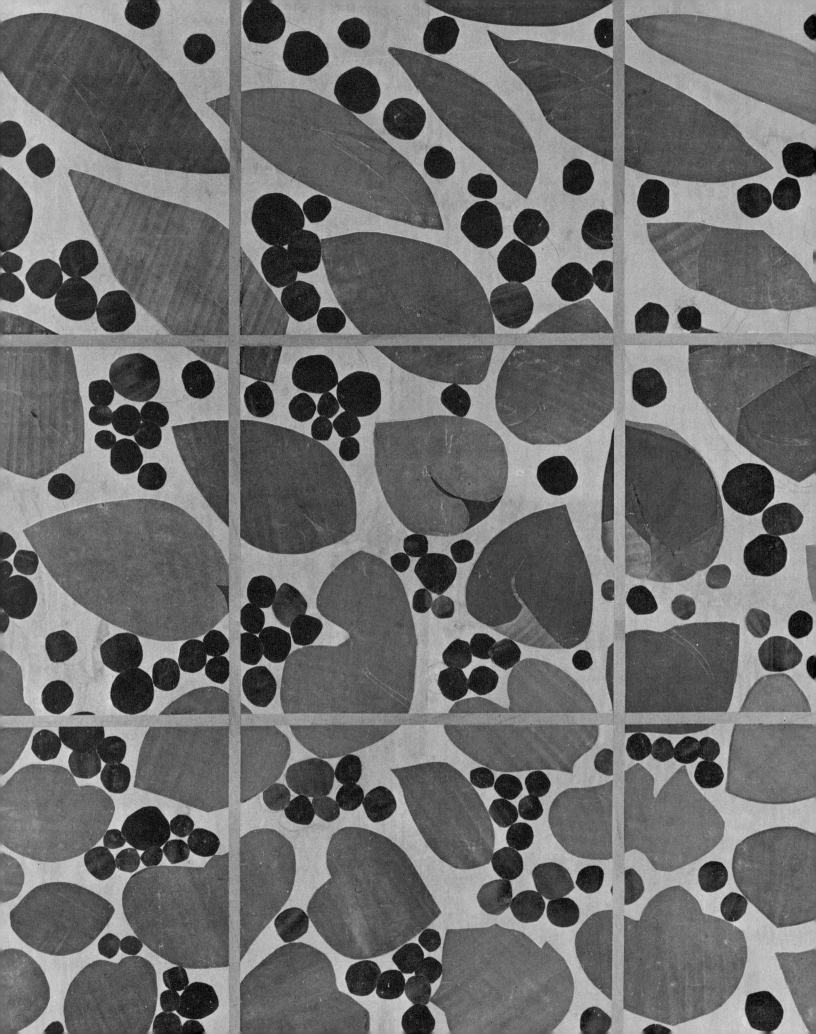

Chapter 5

A Mobilized Army

Blood, the abundant nourisher, is also the great defender, a potent red potion of cells, proteins and enzymes that protects the body from deadly enemies. The white blood cells that constitute the blood's mobilized army fight an endless life-and-death struggle against viruses, bacteria and other microscopic adversaries. Although most bacteria are harmless, and some even beneficial, a few strain the body's system of defense to its limit. One thousand grams of the toxin produced by the botulin bacterium could, in theory, destroy the human race.

The bubonic plague of the fourteenth century is still mankind's grimmest reminder of the power of microorganisms and infectious disease. A third of Europe's population fell in the withering storm of the Black Death. For much of history, man also had to contend with another deadly scourge — smallpox. A smallpox epidemic that killed Mary II, Queen of England, in the seventeenth century moved British historian Thomas Macaulay to write: "The havoc of the [bubonic] plague had been far more rapid: but the plague had visited our shores only once or twice within living memory." Smallpox filled "the churchyards with corpses, tormenting with constant fears all whom it had not yet stricken, leaving on those whose lives it spared the hideous traces of its power, turning the babe into a changeling at which the mother shuddered, and making the eyes and cheeks of the betrothed maiden objects of horror to the lover." Over the course of the eighteenth century, smallpox killed sixty million Europeans. One physician noted that no mother counted her children until they had lived through a wave of the smallpox.

Vaccinations have always been medicine's most effective defense against infectious disease. In rough form, they have existed for centuries. Observation taught man that a brush with a deadly disease left some strange power to protect

Invisible incursions rouse the body's defenders, blood's bitterest denizens. Microscopic trespassers transform them. Sentinels become hordes, a devouring flood in the blood's red river. Blood's army fights life's war.

the stricken from later encounters. Long ago, to combat smallpox, the Chinese powdered bits of dead tissue scraped from the skin of smallpox victims and blew the powder into the noses of healthy people. Greeks and Turks pricked the skin of an uninfected person with a needle just withdrawn from a victim's sore. In India, where vaccination reached a more sophisticated level, physicians extracted pus from mildly infected victims, dried it for a year and used it to vaccinate others. They waited for the weak reaction that followed and used the infected tissues of vaccinated patients to prepare more vaccine. By such device, they lowered the risk of accidentally spreading a virulent strain of the disease.

Lady Mary Wortley Montagu brought Eastern methods of vaccination to England in the early 1700s. Having seen the procedure in Turkey, she recommended that English children be protected in the same way. Known as variolation — from variola, the scientific name for smallpox — Lady Montagu's new method saved the lives of many Europeans in the eighteenth century. At the time she introduced the Turkish practice, one in every fourteen unprotected children in England were dying of smallpox, but variolation was saving ninety-nine of every one hundred treated. Still, it was an imperfect method. Since the procedure required infecting healthy people with live smallpox virus, variolation was occasionally fatal. Breaking the skin with unsterilized needles also spread other infections.

A Country Boy

Safe, modern vaccinations began with the efforts of Edward Jenner, a British country physician. Jenner's genius lay in using cowpox, a less dangerous disease related to smallpox, to produce his vaccine. Raised in rural England, Jenner knew that milkmaids and farmhands who had contracted cowpox were somehow immune to smallpox. In some parts of the countryside, it was even a common practice to make children touch the udders of infected cows so they would contract the disease. Jenner coated the tip of a needle with pus taken from the skin of a woman infected with cowpox. By scratching the arm of a small boy with the needle and infecting him with the

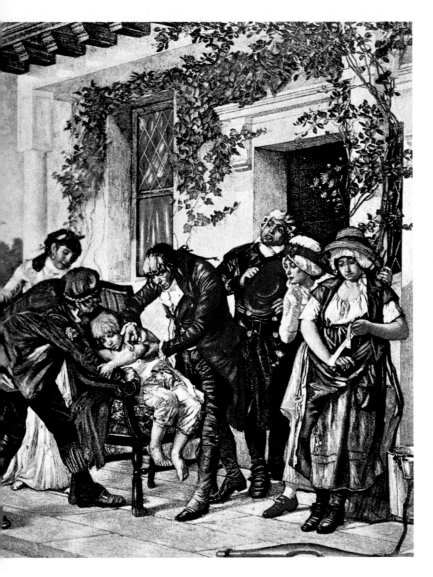

With a small scratch on the arm of eight-year-old James Phipps, British physician Edward Jenner gave man a weapon against infectious disease — a safe method of vaccination. Jenner dipped the tip of his needle in a small cowpox sore on a milkmaid's hand. Cowpox was a mild disease that farmhands sometimes contracted from cattle. By infecting Phipps with cowpox, he safely immunized the boy against a related but much deadlier disease, smallpox.

harmless cowpox virus, he protected the child from smallpox. Jenner's technique remains the basis of all modern vaccinations: the use of weakened or harmless strains of microorganisms to rouse the body's own defenses against future attacks of deadly diseases. Indeed, the scientific name for cowpox is vaccinia, from which the modern word vaccination derives.

Murderous Microbes

Jenner did not know how his vaccination worked. Nor did he know the cause of smallpox. Fifty years would pass before Louis Pasteur and other scientists of the nineteenth century found what they called microbes, the microscopic organisms responsible for infectious disease.

Through his study of diseased tissues, German Rudolph Virchow demonstrated that the cell was the source of health or disease. The integrity of the tissues, the ability of cells to live, grow and reproduce created the steady hum of life. French chemist Louis Pasteur proved that organisms invisible to the naked eye caused putrefaction and disease. His understanding of such microbes eventually led him to develop "attenuation," a method of producing successively weaker generations of microbes for vaccinations. Virchow's countryman Robert Koch isolated and identified the bacteria responsible for tuberculosis and cholera. By the end of the nineteenth century, medicine had vaccines for typhoid fever, tetanus and diphtheria. Before the first decade of the twentieth century had ended, German bacteriologist Paul Ehrlich had developed "606," an effective chemical antagonist to syphilis. His work inaugurated the age of chemotherapy, a word he coined, and presaged still greater medicines to come — penicillin and other antibiotics.

The scientific achievements of the nineteenth century did not stop all deadly infectious diseases. An influenza epidemic swept the world in 1918, leaving fifteen million deaths in its wake. But in less than thirty years, science would make vaccines to control influenza, tuberculosis and yellow fever. Jenner's heirs, improving on his method, have brought many deadly diseases under control in less than a century. In the early 1950s, American physician Jonas Salk developed

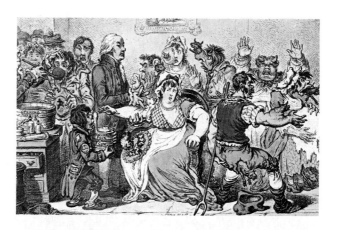

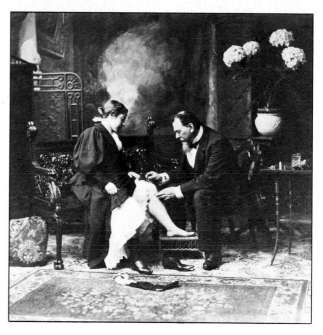

In the early 1800s, cowpox vaccinations were controversial. Diseases from cows, satirists pointed out, could only have unnatural effects, top. But, by the late 1800s, vaccinations were common, above.

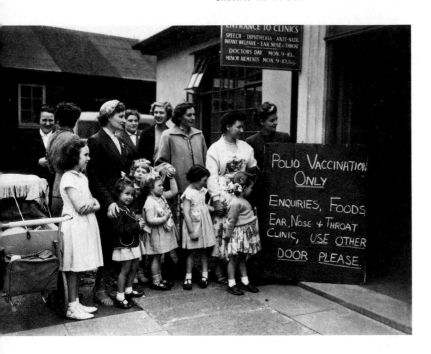

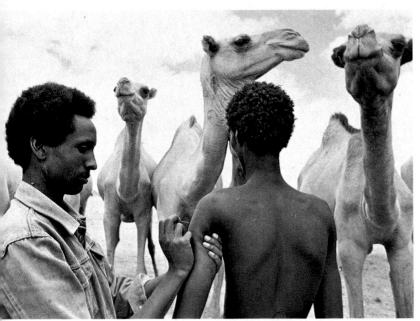

An Ethiopian doctor vaccinates a patient as part of a smallpox eradi-cation program. Vaccinations have vanquished smallpox. The last reported case of the disease occurred in Africa in 1977.

a vaccine for poliomyelitis. Vaccines for measles and rubella (German measles) followed in the 1960s. Most children in the United States are now vaccinated against diphtheria, tetanus, measles, mumps, polio, rubella and whooping cough.

Like the cellular basis of disease, the workings of the body's immune system were still mysteries in the mid-nineteenth century. Scientists knew that blood and tissues were made up of many different components, but they had little sound knowledge of the nature and function of each. The changes that took place in inflamed and pus-filled tissues were largely misunderstood. In 1843, British physician William Addison suggested that the strange white cells found in sores and wounds were the same white cells that circulated in the blood stream. Another Briton, physiologist Augustus Volney Waller, watched these cells squeeze through the walls of capillaries and move to inflamed tissue. In Germany, Jules Cohnheim confirmed these observations and showed conclusively that white blood cells migrated out of the blood stream and into injured tissue. By the 1880s, scientists had also learned that blood had an inexplicable ability to neutralize the toxic chemicals manufactured by some bacteria. Ehrlich demonstrated that blood could build up resistance to potent plant toxins until laboratory animals could survive many times a lethal dose. But what these antitoxins were and how they came about remained unknown.

The White Revolution

Just as it began to be thought that some invisible substance in the blood must be the key to the body's ability to defend itself from microbes, mercurial Russian zoologist Elie Metchnikoff began his own revolution in immunology. The same colorless, wandering cells that Addison, Waller and Cohnheim had implicated in the process of inflammation, Metchnikoff said, were the ones that devoured deadly bacteria. He called them phagocytes, "cell eaters," because they protected the body from disease.

In 1878, Metchnikoff published a report on wandering cells in marine sponges. The cells seemed to crawl through the tissues of the sponges, ingesting bits of food and occasionally

Edward Jenner
Louis Pasteur
Pioneers of Immunology

In 1813, an aging English physician, Edward Jenner, wrote to Napoleon asking that an imprisoned relative be freed. On reading the letter, Napoleon declared, "I can refuse Jenner nothing," and promptly ordered the man released. Although Napoleon had never met Jenner, he was well acquainted with his work. By complying with the request, the French emperor paid tribute to the country doctor who had vanquished smallpox, perhaps the world's most feared disease.

Jenner was an unlikely candidate for such a momentous medical achievement. Though he began practicing medicine in 1773, he was apparently more interested in natural history, winning a fellowship in England's prestigious Royal Society for his work on hedgehogs and cuckoos. Since his youth, however, Jenner had been fascinated by a dairymaid's remark that she could not get smallpox because she had once contracted cowpox, a less debilitating illness normally confined to cattle. In 1796, Jenner scratched matter from a cowpox sore into the arm of an eight-year-old boy. Six weeks later, he inoculated the boy with smallpox virus, but the boy remained healthy. Jenner's method of conferring

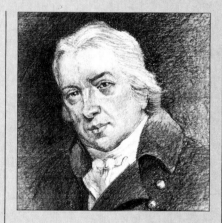

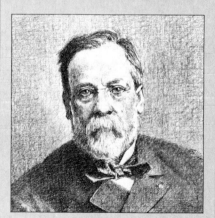

immunity to smallpox spread quickly, drastically cutting the disease's toll. In October 1977, a twenty-three-year-old cook in Somalia had the dubious distinction of becoming the world's last smallpox victim.

Like Jenner, the pioneer French immunologist Louis Pasteur was also influenced by a powerful childhood memory. As a boy, Pasteur saw a man in the agonizing death throes of rabies. He began investigating disease after proving that bacteria were responsible for fermentation. Convinced that microbes also caused disease, he soon isolated the bacteria that caused chicken cholera. After learning to keep the deadly germs alive in broth, he left his laboratory in 1879 for a summer vacation. Upon returning, he inoculated chickens with the cultured bacteria. Remarkably, the birds remained healthy. Later, he inoculated the same chickens with a fresh culture, and again they resisted infection. Puzzled, Pasteur was momentarily silent, and then exclaimed to his colleagues, "Don't you see that these animals have been vaccinated!" During his vacation, the microbes in the broth had grown weak. They roused the chickens' immunological defenses against cholera without causing a fatal infection.

Turning to human diseases, Pasteur developed a rabies vaccine that stopped the disease's progress even after a person became infected. In 1885, he tested the vaccine on a nine-year-old boy, saving his life. The boy became a gatekeeper at the Pasteur Institute. In gratitude to the doctor, he committed suicide rather than open Pasteur's crypt to the invading Nazis in 1940.

A neutrophil, an eosinophil and a monocyte, clockwise from the left, pose together in a capillary. They are the body's three phagocytes, or cell eaters. All three swallow and destroy invading microorganisms.

Magnified more than 6,000 times, red and white blood cells crowd together in an arteriole. Warriors in the body's defense, white blood cells known as leukocytes are round, mobile cells with a rough surface.

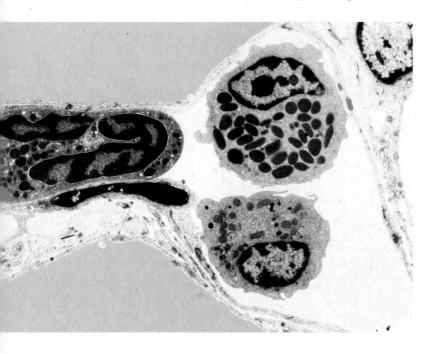

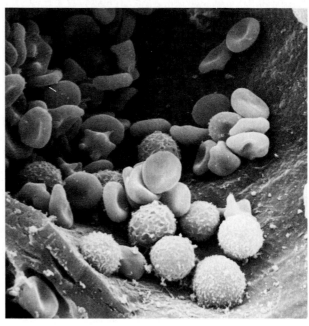

spewing out indigestible particles. In 1882, while studying phagocytes in the transparent larvae of starfish, the realization suddenly struck him that these cells were not digesting the creatures' food. They were destroying microscopic enemies. Eager to prove his theory, Metchnikoff "took several thorns from a rose in order to introduce them beneath the skin of these superb larval starfish, as transparent as water." After a restless night of anticipation, he checked the larvae and found a swarm of phagocytes crowded around the tip of the thorn. Metchnikoff needed nothing more. All immunity from disease, he concluded, came from the exertions of phagocytes.

For more than a decade, the two major views of immunity — one that the blood itself created or possessed products that neutralized toxins and bacteria, and Metchnikoff's notion of cellular defense — contended for supremacy. The succeeding years would prove both sides correct, yet incomplete. The human immune system, scientists now know, is an intricate network of blood, enzyme, cell and hormone, more complex than any nineteenth-century scientist suspected.

Phagocytosis, the process by which a white blood cell devours a bacterium, virus or any kind of biological debris, is a major part of the body's defense system. Five types of white blood cells, or leukocytes, circulate through the blood stream. Three are phagocytes: neutrophils, eosinophils and monocytes. Although related to neutrophils and eosinophils, the fourth type of white blood cell, the basophil, is not a phagocyte. It does not devour other cells but, rather, plays an important role in inflammation and allergic reactions. The fifth type of white blood cell, the lymphocyte, is the key to the body's defense in another branch of the immune system.

The Foot Soldiers

Neutrophils, eosinophils and basophils display tiny granules in their cytoplasm, or cell fluid. These granules, filled with potent chemicals and active proteins called enzymes, give the three cells the name granulocytes. Like monocytes, lymphocytes and all other blood cells, granulocytes are born in the bone marrow. Neutrophils live only five or six days, eosinophils perhaps twice as long. Neutrophils reach full maturity in the bone marrow, which stores billions of them in tiny sinuses, where they wait to be released into the blood stream in response to infection. The bone marrow of a 150-pound man produces roughly 100 billion neutrophils a day. They are

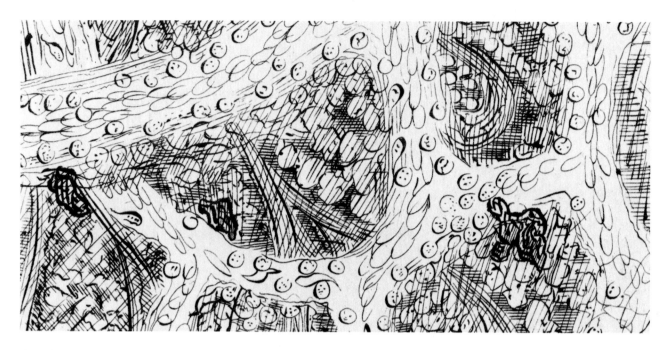

the foot soldiers of the body's immunological army, and they perish in great numbers in the war against disease.

Released from bone marrow, the neutrophils travel to the body's tissues, where they await invasion. They spend only about six hours in the blood stream. Most neutrophils in the blood stream are not actually circulating. At any time, about two-thirds can be found clinging to the inner surfaces of blood vessels. On solid ground, like a capillary wall, neutrophils and all other white blood cells move like amoebas. They stretch out a pseudopod, or foot, and slowly drag their fluid bodies over it. Repeating the process again and again, they ripple through tissues and along capillary walls. Some white blood cells can crawl three times their own length in a minute.

From inside capillary walls, neutrophils and monocytes squeeze through blood vessels and into tissues by a motion known as diapedesis. Through pores between the cells of capillary walls, a white blood cell extends a fingerlike projection, much like a pseudopod, from its soft body. With part of its cell membrane on both sides of the capillary, the neutrophil or monocyte slowly oozes out. Once outside the capillary, it begins its amoeboid march through the tissues.

Bacteria, dying tissues, clotting blood and other cells exude chemicals that inexorably draw white blood cells toward the site of an invasion. This phenomenon is chemotaxis. When foreign matter breaches the skin, proteins in the blood and intercellular fluid also cling to the bacteria or toxins, making them especially attractive to neutrophils. Many foreign particles also bear a rough surface and a strong electric charge, uncommon characteristics in the body's living tissue.

When a neutrophil meets an invading bacterium, the struggle begins in earnest. The neutrophil extends pseudopods out and around the invading cell, surrounding it in a capsule called a phagosome. When the neutrophil has completely engulfed the invader, the phagosome breaks free of the neutrophil's outer cell membrane and floats like a bubble in the cell's cytoplasm. Inside the neutrophil, a granule filled with powerful enzymes eventually comes in contact with the outer surface of the phagosome. The two chambers fuse, and the granule spews its contents into the phagosome, disintegrating the bacterium. The neutrophils also have chambers that synthesize hydrogen peroxide, a chemical that burns up tough bacterial membranes. In defending the body, neutrophils die by the billions. Some bac-

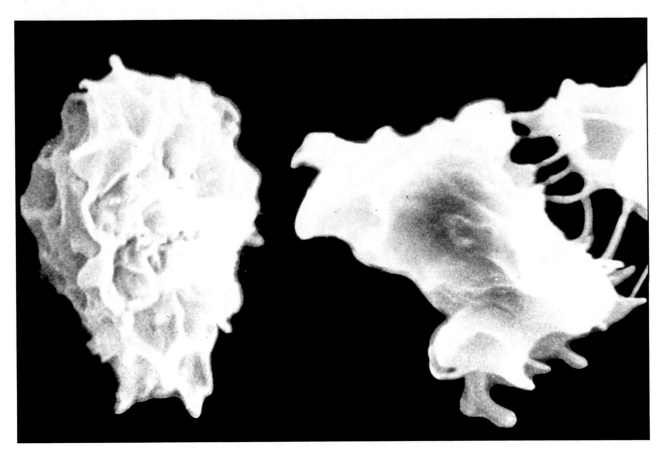

teria are formidable enemies, capable of destroying the body's troops. Neutrophils themselves can endure pitched battle only so long. Having ingested as few as five or as many as fifty bacteria, a neutrophil will have exhausted its store of granules. It succumbs to the toxins of the invaders and its own digestive enzymes.

Storm Troopers

While neutrophils — in part by the weight of their sheer number — carry on the struggle against microscopic invaders, monocytes assume another posture in the common defense. When they enter invaded tissues, monocytes undergo a remarkable transformation. Swelling five or even ten times their original size, monocytes become macrophages, large phagocytic cells able to devour a hundred invaders and still survive.

Monocytes in the blood stream have a limited ability to digest foreign invaders. Like neutro-

phils, they cling to the walls of blood vessels, squeeze through capillaries and crawl through blood vessels and tissues. Scientists suspect that monocytes and macrophages also can produce at least one of a group of substances collectively known as colony-stimulating factor (CSF), which prompts marrow to produce more monocytes and neutrophils. But compared to macrophages, monocytes are still raw recruits, unready for a pitched immunological battle.

The macrophage's simplest role is that of a huge, tireless phagocyte with an almost insatiable appetite. Macrophage means "big eater," and this special cell is well named. Some macrophages live for years. Instead of being destroyed by their own digestive enzymes, they can empty the contents of their phagosomes into surrounding tissue. There, neutrophils or other macrophages continue the struggle. In a battle against a particularly large or resilient foe, several macro-

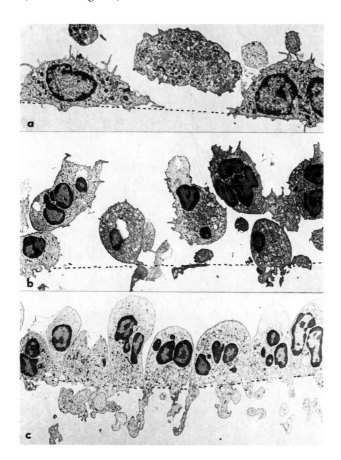

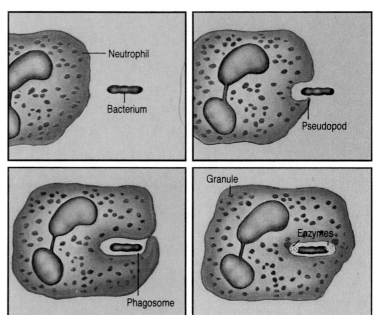

As a neutrophil meets an invading bacterium, it stretches out pseudopods, trapping the enemy in a chamber called a phagosome. Inside the neutrophil, granules filled with corrosive enzymes fuse with the membrane of the phagosome and dump their contents into the minute prison, destroying the bacterium. Immunologists call this process of consuming aliens phagocytosis.

phages can also fuse together to form a huge cell with many nuclei, called a giant cell. Giant cells are rich in lysosomes, small pockets of potent enzymes similar to the granules in neutrophils.

Macrophages take up residence in different tissues of the body. Some wander through skin or intestine, others send out small branches, called dendrites, to anchor themselves in one place. Alerted to an infection, however, wandering macrophages descend on injured tissue to consume invaders, while fixed macrophages can free themselves from their normal posts and migrate to the site of invasion.

Macrophages line the lungs, intestines and many other organs. In different parts of the body, they bear different names: dendritic macrophages are found in lymph nodes, Kupffer's cells in the liver, tissue histiocytes in connective tissue surrounding skin and muscle. Unlike neutrophils, macrophages can reproduce, multiplying

Jonas Salk

Conqueror of Polio

From his sequestered office overlooking the Pacific Ocean, Jonas Salk sustains an abiding faith in mankind's capacity to create a better world. "I think we're generally programmed to solve problems we create," he maintains, "even though it appears we're on the verge of autodestruction." Salk's words carry unusual authority, for any survey of gifted problem-solvers would almost certainly include his name. Though Salk continues to decode biological puzzles at the California research center that bears his name, he is best remembered as the scientific hero who conquered polio.

Born in 1914 in a New York tenement, Salk abandoned a career as a practicing physician to conduct his own research. Asked why he pursued $1,500- and $2,500-a-year fellowships instead of a lucrative medical practice, he replied, "Why did Mozart compose music?"

Salk's chance to compose a brilliant scientific score came in 1947. Frustrated with the progress of his career, he accepted a position at the University of Pittsburgh, where he would head a project to study polio viruses. At the time, polio struck thousands of Americans each year, mainly children. Many died, but far more were crippled for life.

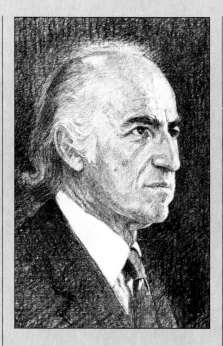

In extreme cases, even the muscles that control breathing became paralyzed. A person so affected was confined to a grim device known popularly as the iron lung. Among polio's most prominent victims was Franklin Delano Roosevelt, who contracted the disease in 1921. Born too early to take advantage of Salk's discovery, Roosevelt remained a cripple for the rest of his life.

After confirming that among hundreds of strains of polio viruses, only three varieties threatened man, Salk began research on potential vaccines. Attempts in the 1930s to develop an effective polio vaccine had met with disaster, and several children died in the early tests. In isolating his vaccine, Salk proceeded on the assumption that viruses could be killed but still stimulate the production of antibodies. Selecting the three highly virulent strains, Salk killed them in a formaldehyde solution. Because some viruses might survive this lethal bath by hiding in solid particles, he thoroughly filtered the mixture. Testing this vaccine on rhesus monkeys, he found dramatically increased antibody levels. For his first test on humans, Salk vaccinated children already crippled by the disease. Again, antibody levels soared. Later, Salk remarked, "When you inoculate children with a polio vaccine, you don't sleep well for two or three months."

Salk's vaccine was ready for nationwide testing in 1954. Nearly 450,000 children lined up in schools, armories and gymnasiums around the country to receive their vaccinations. In April 1955, the results were announced. The vaccine was proven 60 percent effective against type I polio, and 90 percent effective against types II and III. Salk became an overnight celebrity, and within seven years polio was virtually wiped out in the United States.

their numbers at their immunological outposts while they wait for neutrophils to pour in.

The macrophage's role extends beyond engulfing microorganisms. They are also the body's scavengers, devouring diseased or battered red blood cells, exhausted neutrophils, bits of dead tissue and other debris. The speed at which some macrophages ingest invaders almost defies detection. Slow-motion photography of macrophages in the liver reveals that they consume bacteria in less than one one-hundredth of a second. Like neutrophils, they surround their prey with pseudopods and encapsulate them in a digestive chamber. Lysosomes then eject their contents into the digestive capsule to destroy the invader. Even indigestible materials come to an end inside macrophages. What macrophages cannot destroy, they sometimes preserve. They swallow up some indestructible invaders and imprison them.

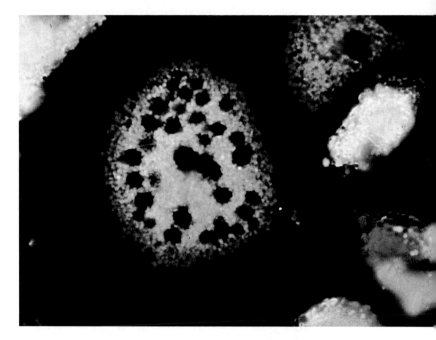

A Call to Arms

Macrophages, neutrophils and other white blood cells respond to inflammation, the body's call to arms. Attacked by bacteria, toxins or viruses, tissue releases histamine and other substances that begin inflammation. These messengers dilate capillaries and venules and make the walls of blood vessels more permeable to white blood cells, fluid and clotting proteins.

As the clotting factors in blood leak into the tissues near the site of an infection, they begin to seal off the area to prevent the spread of toxins and bacteria. Other by-products of tissue damage leak back through the blood stream and signal bone marrow to release stored white blood cells. The number of neutrophils in the blood stream can multiply five times in the first few hours of a serious infection. The capillary walls become stickier to trap passing white blood cells and the inflamed tissues beckon phagocytes. Tissue macrophages at the invasion site might liberate CSF to increase production of neutrophils and monocytes in bone marrow. Macrophages near the site reproduce, dividing into larger colonies of hungry phagocytes. As battle progresses, billions of phagocytes perish. Depleted of their digestive enzymes, the fallen white blood cells mingle on the field of battle with defeated microorganisms,

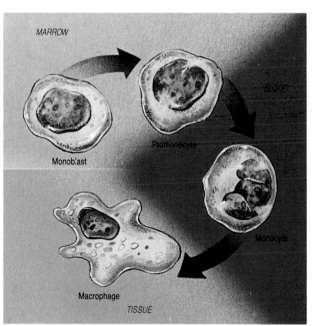

In the bone marrow, monoblasts and promonocytes mature into monocytes, which enter the blood. An assault by microorganisms calls monocytes from blood to tissue, where they grow into macrophages.

Inflammation is the body's call to arms. Invading microorganisms cause mast cells to release histamine and other substances, which dilate blood vessels and make capillary walls stickier and more permeable.

Fluids and proteins leak into tissue. Passing white blood cells cluster on capillary walls. By a motion known as diapedesis, the defenders then squeeze through tiny pores into invaded tissue.

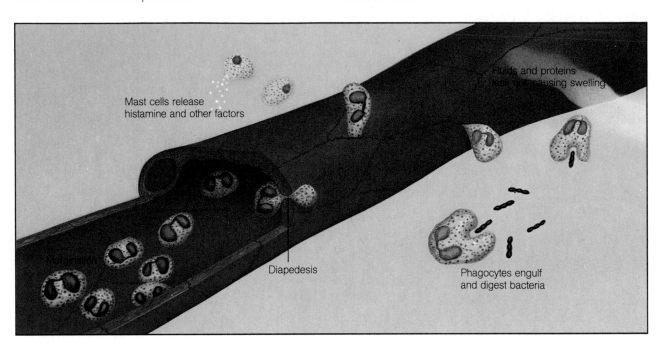

Mast cells release histamine and other factors

Fluids and proteins leak out, causing swelling

Margination

Diapedesis

Phagocytes engulf and digest bacteria

bits of dead tissue and other debris of immunological warfare. A small patch of inflamed tissue might appear, the signal of a successful defense.

Phagocytes are the infantry of the immune system. Many lower animals have only phagocytes, some internal enzymes and the barrier of their skins to protect them. In man, these same elements present a potent deterrent to invading microorganisms. Sweat glands secrete chemicals highly toxic to many microscopic trespassers. Mucous membranes in the nose and throat and acids in the stomach frustrate the growth of bacteria. Some proteins in blood — the properdin proteins — can bind to the outside of certain bacteria and begin a chemical chain reaction that destroys the invaders. Phagocytes are always ready to swarm indiscriminately over any invaders that breach the outer defenses. But in man and other mammals, these defenses are not enough. They are merely the simplest methods of defense in a system so complex that most of what medicine knows about its inner workings has been discovered only in the last thirty years.

The response of phagocytes to foreign invaders is nonspecific immunity. But the human body possesses immunological defenses designed to seek specific bacteria and viruses with uncanny accuracy. The lymphocyte is the fundamental cellular unit of the specific immune system. About 25 percent of circulating white blood cells are lymphocytes. At any given time, the vast majority of these cells are not crawling through the blood stream but waiting in the body's tissues, especially lymphatic tissue. Lymphocytes derive their name from lymph, the clear fluid that transports them in vast numbers.

The lymphatic system is a kind of secondary circulatory system, complementing the blood stream. White blood cells, food, fluid and oxygen flow through the blood stream on their way to the body's tissues. But to reach individual cells, provisions in the blood must leave the capillaries and enter the interstitial fluid, a clear, colorless liquid that bathes all body cells. Some of this fluid collects in tiny ducts, lymphatic channels, that wind near skin, muscle, bone and organs throughout the body. The normal contraction of muscles squeezes lymph in these channels toward the chest. There, large lymphatic ducts empty into veins near the heart. Fluid, proteins and lymphocytes pour into the blood stream, completing a long circuit from the blood, through the tissues, along the lymphatic pathway and back to the blood.

In the defense of the body, the lymphatic system picks up bacteria and other invaders that penetrate the skin or capillaries and carries them to special lymphatic tissues. Spleen, tonsils, lymph nodes, adenoids, and bone marrow are all important outposts for lymphocytes, which lie in wait for hostile microorganisms.

Assassins with Magic Bullets

Although small, sluggish, devoid of granules or lysosomes and powerless to devour a foreign cell, lymphocytes are deadly immunological weapons. Their attack on an invader is more subtle than a phagocyte's, but no less effective. Phagocytes devour whatever alien substances cross their path, or die in the attempt. A lymphocyte seeks its particular foe, a bit of foreign tissue that it recognizes from among all others, and destroys it with the single-minded intensity of an assassin.

Lymphocytes divide into two major classes, B lymphocytes, or B cells, and T lymphocytes, or T cells. Under a microscope, they look alike. But their roles are different and complementary. B cells produce antibodies, the immune system's magic bullets that seek out specific invaders and trigger a process that leads to the invaders' destruction. Antibodies in blood and lymph constitute humoral immunity, so named because body fluids, long called humors, transport antibodies to the battlefields of immunological warfare. Antibodies are proteins, not cells. Unlike phagocytes or lymphocytes, they cannot crawl to the site of an invasion. T cells, too, respond only to specific microorganisms. Instead of producing antibodies, the three varieties of T cells perform other tasks. Some attack the invader directly with potent chemicals. Others prod B cells to produce antibodies. The third variety helps regulate the immune response, protecting the body from the excesses of its own defense. The work of T cells is called cell-mediated immunity.

Any substance that elicits a response from B or T cells is an antigen. Antigens are innumerable. Bacteria, toxins, viruses, living and dead tissue and bits of organic and inorganic debris can all trigger an immune response. Bacteria, among the deadliest antigens, carry proteins and sugars on their cell membranes that label them as accurate-

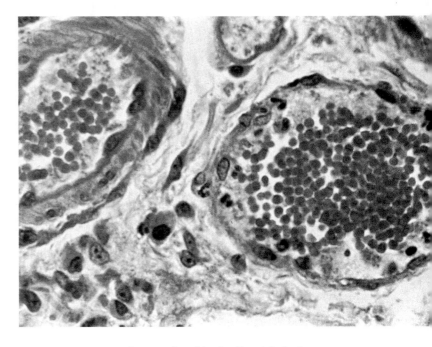

Large white blood cells with dark nuclei ring hundreds of smaller red blood cells pouring through an artery. Inflammation snares white blood cells on vessel walls, a process called margination.

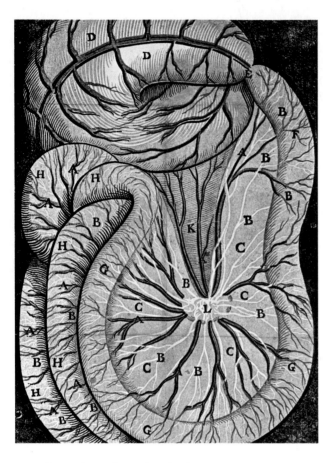

Lymphatic channels in the small intestines, called lacteals, were one of the subjects of the first colored anatomical drawings, published in 1627 by Italian physician and anatomist Gaspar Aselli.

ly as a fingerprint labels a man. Some of these proteins and sugars, called antigenic determinants, mark the bacteria as foes. All living tissue displays markers that could activate a B or T cell, even the tissues of the human body. Individual B and T cells are genetically programmed to recognize their foe among the millions that might invade the human body. They exist to distinguish the body's own tissues and other harmless or beneficial substances from potentially deadly aliens, to separate the "self" from "nonself."

Both kinds of lymphocytes derive from stem cells in the bone marrow, as do all blood cells. Stem cells produce immature lymphocytes that later mature into B or T cells. In the fetus, under the influence of thymic hormones, some lymphocytes migrate to the thymus gland, a small pink bag of tissue behind the breastbone. Many cells processed in the thymus, T cells, journey to the spleen, lymph nodes and other lymphatic tissue. The remaining cells in the thymus and many of the T cells newly arrived in the lymphatic tissue are themselves capable of reproducing and maintaining the supply of T cells. Thymic hormones influence the development of all T cells, and may be partially responsible for determining the later identity of immature T cells.

Immunologists remain uncertain about the exact location of the processing center for B cells in the human body. Antibody-producing lymphocytes in all animals are called B cells because researchers first found uncommitted lymphocytes maturing into antibody producers in the bursa of Fabricius, a small patch of intestinal tissue in chickens. But mammals have no corresponding intestinal tissue. Only recently have some immunologists come to believe that bone marrow is the center for processing B cells. Many B cells freed from the bone marrow, like T cells, circulate through blood and lymph, eventually settling in lymphatic tissues. B and T cells that do not encounter their special foes die in the blood stream or peripheral tissues. Those that meet their enemy prepare for later encounters. Waiting for the reappearance of an antigen, some lymphocytes circulate through the body for years.

Of the millions of lymphocytes in a lymph gland, only a few might respond to a particular

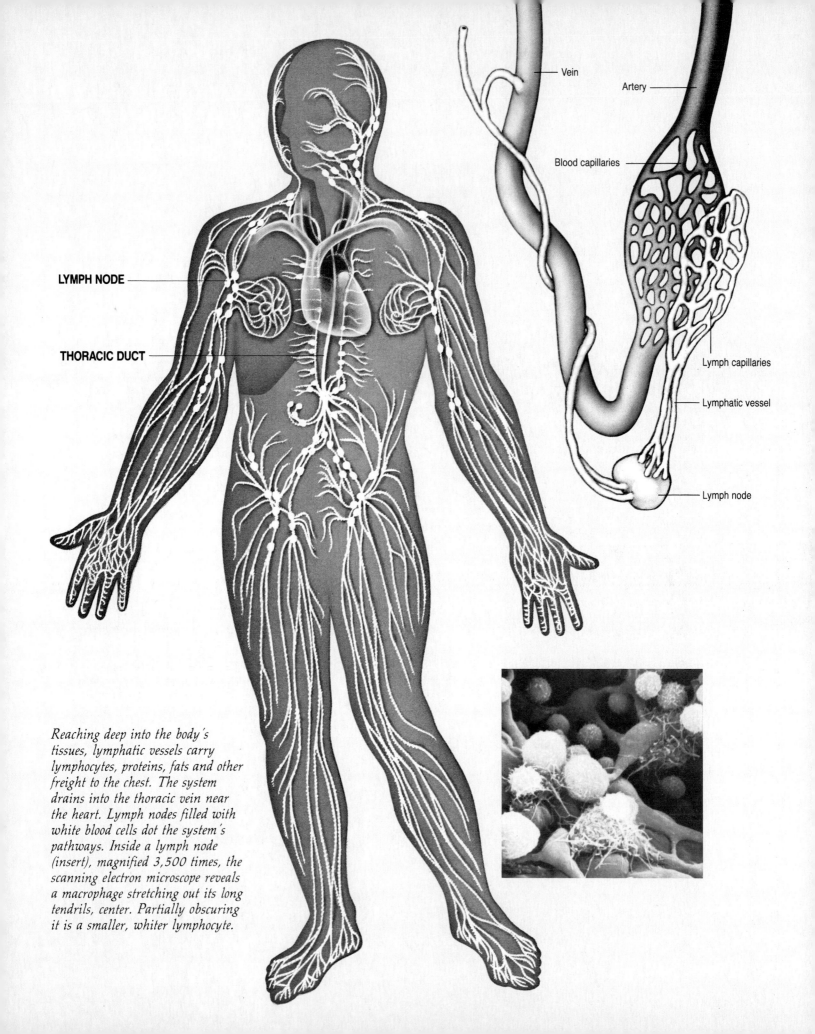

Vein

Artery

Blood capillaries

LYMPH NODE

Lymph capillaries

THORACIC DUCT

Lymphatic vessel

Lymph node

Reaching deep into the body's tissues, lymphatic vessels carry lymphocytes, proteins, fats and other freight to the chest. The system drains into the thoracic vein near the heart. Lymph nodes filled with white blood cells dot the system's pathways. Inside a lymph node (insert), magnified 3,500 times, the scanning electron microscope reveals a macrophage stretching out its long tendrils, center. Partially obscuring it is a smaller, whiter lymphocyte.

antigen. But all lymphocytes that respond to a given antigen form what is known as a clone. Lymphocytes in blood, lymph and tissue reproduce after an encounter with their specific antigen to increase the size of their clones.

Guided Missiles

Against most bacteria, the immune system's most effective weapon is the antibody, the B cell's remarkable creation. Antibodies, proteins that circulate in the blood stream, are called gamma globulins or immunoglobulins. Five varieties of antibodies exist: immunoglobulin A (IgA), IgD, IgE, IgG and IgM. IgA is found mainly in the body's mucous membranes, where it intercepts antigens in the nose and throat. IgE binds to certain antigens to cause allergic reactions. Little is known of IgD's task. The largest antibody, IgM, and IgG, the most common, play the major role in attacking many bacteria and other antigens.

Antibodies consist of two chains of amino acids, the building blocks of proteins. Shaped like a **Y**, antibodies have two long heavy amino acid chains joined side by side, to form the trunk of the **Y**. At one end, the heavy chains bend slightly outward, forming the branches of the **Y**. Along these diverging branches lie two short, light chains. At the end of all four chains of every antibody is a tiny segment, called the variable portion, that binds to antigens with the perfect fit of a key in a lock. Any B cell or clone of B cells produces antibodies keyed to one specific antigen, although a large bacterium might have many antigenic proteins or sugars on its surface. The trunk of the antibody and the lower parts of both branches make up its constant portion. The antibody's constant portion identifies its class, such as IgG or IgM, and enables the antibody to initiate an enzymatic chain reaction in the blood stream that destroys its antigen.

B cells carry about one hundred thousand identical surface receptors on their cell membranes. In a way, the receptors are replicas of the antibodies that the cell will eventually produce. When cell and antigen meet, the antigen binds to the cell's surface receptors. Immediately, the B cell enlarges, changing its shape and appearance. Most of the B cells in any clone go on to form

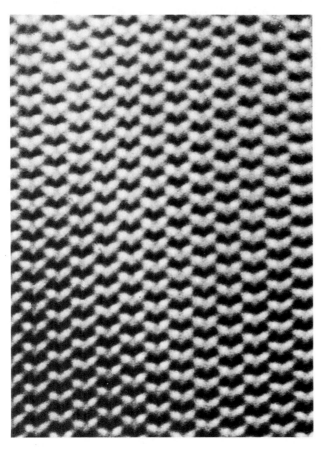

Crystalized antibodies magnified 1,450,000 times show their Y-shaped structure. Repeated photographic exposures of a smaller pattern of antibodies yielded the fabric of crystals shown above. Antibodies consist of two long, heavy chains of amino acids joined side-by-side and flanked on one end by two shorter, lighter chains. Bends in the heavy chains give antibodies their characteristic Y shape.

Small molecules of protein or sugar identify bacteria and other antigens as invaders. Antibodies recognize these antigenic determinants and lock onto them with a perfect, minute, three-dimensional grip.

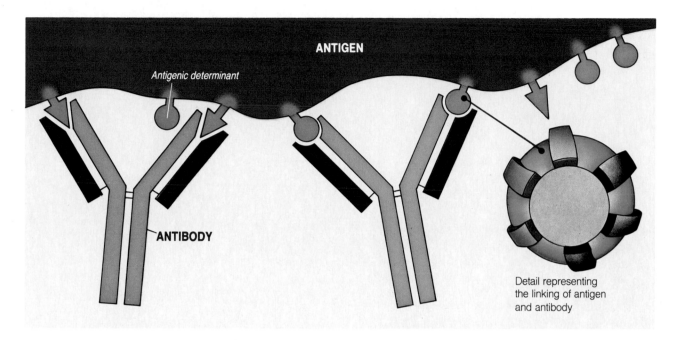

ANTIGEN

Antigenic determinant

ANTIBODY

Detail representing the linking of antigen and antibody

plasma cells, the production plants of antibodies. One lymphocyte can multiply wildly into hundreds of plasma cells over the course of a few days. When the plasma cells mature, they begin manufacturing antibodies — roughly 2,000 every second. Plasma cells produce IgM antibodies first, and then switch to make IgG antibodies for the remainder of their few days of life.

The stimulated lymphocytes that do not become plasma cells prepare the body for the next encounter with the antigen by transforming into memory cells and multiplying rapidly. Memory cells expand the size of a clone of lymphocytes and enable the body to mount a more powerful response to any antigen it meets more than once. Memory cells are the key to vaccination. A small, harmless exposure to dead or weakened bacteria can prompt a clone to form both antibodies and memory cells. Immunologists call this the primary response. Should a virulent form of the bacteria find its way into the body, the pool of waiting memory cells will launch a secondary response — a flood of antibodies usually massive enough to overwhelm the invasion.

Many memory cells take up permanent residence in lymph nodes, the gastrointestinal tract or the spleen. Some, however, begin the long cir-

cuit through the lymphatic system and the blood stream, where they join other circulating lymphocytes on guard for their chosen antigen. The continuous movement of memory cells spreads sensitized lymphocytes throughout the body to man the walls of the self.

Each of the three T cells — killer, helper and suppressor — also react to its initial encounter with invaders by forming memory cells and active cells. Often, a single strain of bacteria will trigger the proliferation of both B and T cells. Immunologists have not yet been able to detect the crucial receptors on the T cells' membranes that permit the cells to recognize their foes.

Antibodies persist in the blood stream for only a few weeks before breaking down. But just like B memory cells, the memory killer, helper and suppressor T cells can live for years. The average lifespan of a T cell is roughly four-and-one-half years. Researchers speculate that some might live for as long as twenty years. The assault of antibodies is the immune system's main defense against acute bacterial infection. T cells destroy invading fungal cells, cancerous cells, surgically transplanted tissue and wounded cells harboring viruses or bacteria inside their cell membranes, where antibodies cannot reach them.

113

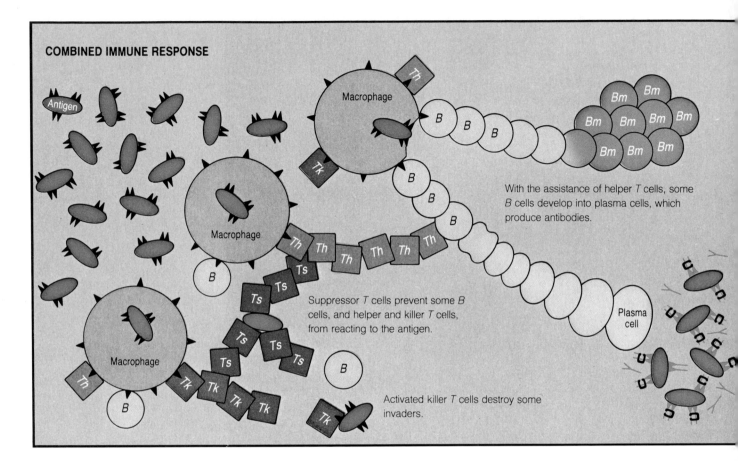

COMBINED IMMUNE RESPONSE

With the assistance of helper *T* cells, some *B* cells develop into plasma cells, which produce antibodies.

Suppressor *T* cells prevent some *B* cells, and helper and killer *T* cells, from reacting to the antigen.

Activated killer *T* cells destroy some invaders.

The combined immune response is a concerted struggle in the body's defense. Macrophages, neutrophils, B cells and suppressor (Ts), killer (Tk) and helper (Th) cells all play a role. The macrophages devour invading antigens, such as bacteria, and present evidence of the attack to lymphocytes. B cells and helper and killer T cells swarming around the macrophages recognize the invaders and begin to multiply. Suppressor T cells seem to take their cue directly from antigens. All four varieties of lymphocytes produce active cells and memory cells. B memory cells (Bm) form a cluster, top center. The interaction of all the cells as they multiply prompts a full-scale immune response, destroying the invaders.

Phagocytes and lymphocytes are the major weapons in the body's defense, but their interaction with invaders and each other brings still other forces into play. Microorganisms pouring in through a wound might first encounter a few B and T cells, macrophages or neutrophils. The combined cell forces are sufficient to begin the immune response, but they are not strong enough to halt the invasion. Activated phagocytes, lymphocytes and injured tissue release a flood of chemical signals that start the process of inflammation and step up the manufacture and release of phagocytes from the bone marrow. This irresistible lure of chemotaxis draws macrophages, neutrophils and lymphoctyes to the site of the invasion. Any antibodies already in the area lock onto their predestined foes.

The binding of antibody to antigen initiates another explosion of chemical activity called the complement reaction. When an IgM or two IgG

THE COMPLEMENT SYSTEM

*Complement proteins are a nine-
member squad of saboteurs. Two adjacent IgG antibodies on a bacte-
or other antigen trigger the comp
ment reaction. The first complem
protein, C1, bridges the two ant
ies. One of its subunits, C1s, sp
two more complement proteins, C
and C2. Bits of the fractured proteins, now active enzymes, bind t
surface of the bacterium. Throug
the complement reaction, fragmer
enzymes drift off in blood or lym
perform other tasks in the comm
defense, such as summoning phag
cytes and promoting inflammatio*

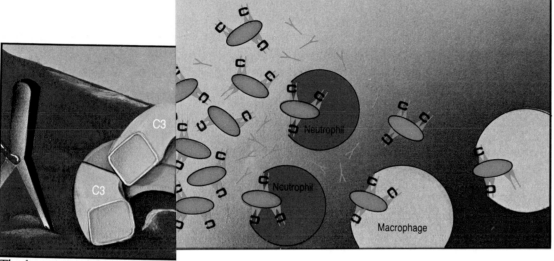

Antibodies released from plasma cells pour into the blood stream
and coat the invading bacteria. Two *IgG* antibodies clinging to
adjacent sites on a bacterium activate complement enzymes (C),
which destroy the invaders. Antibodies, complement enzymes and
chemicals released from damaged tissues also attract macrophages and neutrophils to devour bacteria.

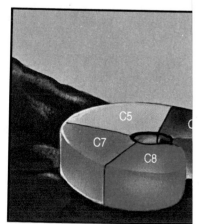

*The fragments of C4 and C2 lock
split the next complement enzyme,
enzymes cleave C5.*

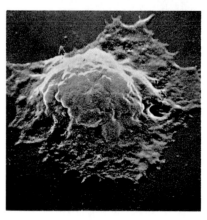

*Carrying C6 and C7, the C5 enzy
on the bacterium, where C8 and C
zymes begin to gnaw at the bacteri*

antibodies combine with a specific antigen, a
change in the shape of the antibody molecules
exposes a hidden portion of their surface to the
surrounding fluid. This change activates complement proteins in the blood stream. A cascade of
chemical interactions fractures some of the nine
different proteins in the complement system,
transforming the fragments into active enzymes.
A few of these enzymes bind to the antigen near
the site of the antigen-antibody complex.

Complement enzymes burn holes in the tough
outer membranes of many bacteria. Once the
membrane of an alien has been penetrated, it explodes. Bits of complement proteins can also
neutralize some viruses, while other fragments
attach to antigens and label the invaders enemies,
making them especially susceptible to phagocytosis. The destruction of the invaders liberates
still more chemicals and biological debris into the
tissues, reinforcing the immune response. But the

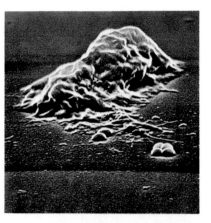

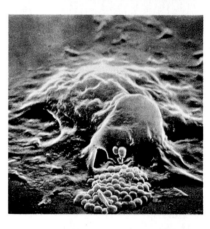

*Like a nightmare lurching to life,
a macrophage devours a colony of
bacteria. Although the body's huge
defenders seem sluggish and shape-
less, macrophages engulf trespassers
in a fraction of a second.*

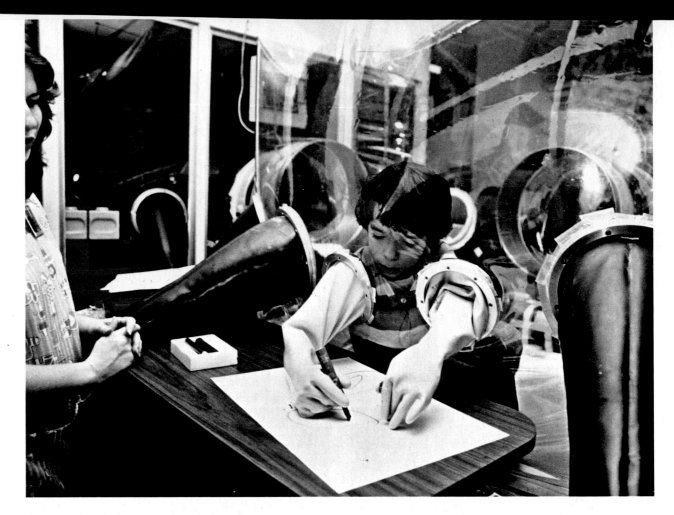

Although they are protein[...] much smaller than bacter[...] bodies can unite two inva[...] This clumping process, kn[...] agglutination, makes bact[...] targets for phagocytes.

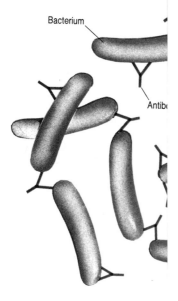

Bacterium

Antib[...]

destructive powers of
have inherent limits th
ning amok. With rare
proteins only bind to
antibodies, protecting
effects of the powerf[...]
enzymes are themselve
to destroying foreign c
enzymes attract phago[...]
chemicals and dying ba

As they activate th
antibodies clinging to a[...]
er identical antigens or
teins and antibodies. Th
agglutination, produces
and antigens, easy targ
neutrophils. Coated wi
gens normally small en[...]
become too large and h[...]
fluids. They settle out
stick to vessel walls,
hungry phagocytes.

In addition to con
macrophages process th
tein that signal the id[...]
concentrated form, wh
call "superantigen," the[...]

Some T cells also secrete a lymphokine that activates other T cells of the same clone, even those far removed from the site of an invasion. This transfer factor seems to hold the power to transform a local T cell response into a widespread reaction throughout the body, in advance of the spread of an antigen.

With a successful defense, the immune response gradually winds down. Different factors curtail the battle. As the microscopic invaders disappear, the stimulus to fight declines. High levels of antibodies in the blood stream also slow the creation of more antibodies, and suppressor T cells constantly monitor and adjust the manufacture of antibodies, counteracting the efforts of the helper T cells and maintaining the defensive response at the proper level.

One theory of the workings of the immune system holds that it is an intricate network of antibodies, B cells and T cells that react not only with antigens but with each other. Just as every antibody has a region coded to interact with an antigen, it also displays a particular arrangement of amino acids somewhere on its surface that identifies it. Researchers call this arrangement its idiotype. In a way similar to their interaction with antigens, antibodies and lymphocytes with corresponding idiotypes interact with each other and either suppress or activate the immune response. A massive invasion of outside antigens disrupts the calm, steady state of the immune system, until the foreign antigens are destroyed. Then, according to the network theory, the parts of the immune system return to a delicate balance, preserving a state of perpetual readiness and single-minded hostility to invaders.

The remarkable power of the immune system is perhaps best illustrated by the havoc that accompanies its failure. If the bone marrow stops producing neutrophils, bacterial invasions can lead to agranulocytosis. This condition ends the steady skirmishing of bacteria and neutrophils and allows the invaders to multiply and mount an irresistible attack.

The Field Undefended

B cells, T cells or both are absent in some rare genetic diseases. Because destroying alien tissue is the special province of T cells, children lacking T cells cannot reject transplanted tissue from other people. But neither can they adequately defend themselves against viruses, mutant cells from their own bodies and other antigens, since helper T cells are crucial in stimulating B cells to make antibodies. A lack of effective B cells and antibodies, called agammaglobulinemia, leaves a child unable to mount a full-scale immune attack on many virulent bacteria but does not prevent the rejection of transplants and the destruction of some antigens by T cells. Severe T cell deficiencies and agammaglobulinemia are often fatal early in life. Antibiotics offer some protection. Passive immunity, the technique of injecting antibodies or sensitized T cells from one person into the blood stream of another, can protect people with immunological deficiencies for a few days or weeks. For the first six to nine months of life, before the immune system is fully prepared to recognize and destroy deadly emissaries from the outside world, the transfer of the mother's antibodies to her fetus is what enables it to survive. During a child's first year, passive immunity gives way to active immunity as the infant's own lymphocytes encounter their predestined foes and develop into active, competent sentries in the body's defense.

Civilian Casualties

Not all the quirks of the immune system are as rare as agranulocytosis or agammaglobulinemia. Allergies, common maladjustments of the immune response, affect about thirty-seven million people in the United States. Almost any substance could conceivably provoke an allergic response in someone. Dust, milk, molds, eggs and pollen are common instigators of allergies. No matter what the particular allergy, in an allergic reaction the body mounts an immune response out of proportion to the apparent destructiveness of the invader. The watchful defenses of the body lash back at a harmless irritation.

Allergies seem to be hereditary. The most common types, hay fever and asthma, are immediate reactions. They show unusually high quantities of IgE antibodies in the blood, from 10 to 100 times higher than normal. Discovered in 1966, IgE antibodies are now a vital diagnostic sign of many allergies. Although IgE antibodies are considered immunoglobulins along with IgG, IgM and other antibodies, allergists often call them by the special name reagins. The antigens that elicit a response from IgE antibodies are allergens.

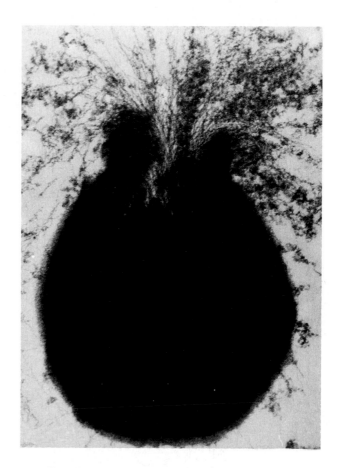

Its cell wall gashed by antibiotics, a bacterium explodes. Antibiotics are the immune system's most effective medical ally. But passive immunity, transfusions of antibodies and lymphocytes, can also stave off disease.

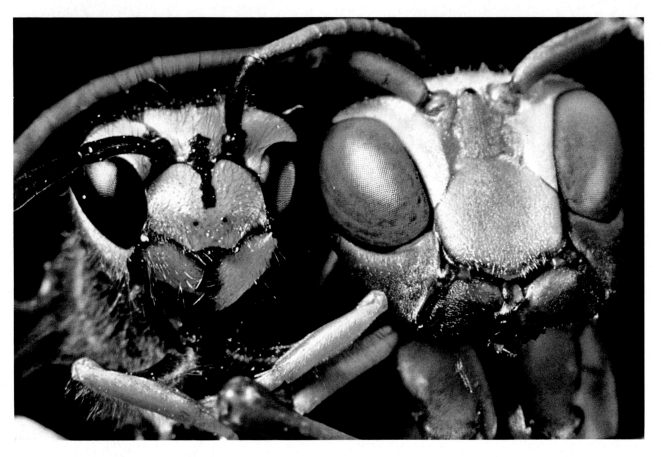

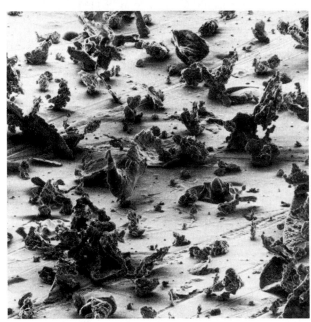

Allergies develop from repeated exposures to allergens over a period of time. Like a vaccination gone awry, the body produces greater numbers of IgE antibodies with successive exposures to the allergen. Allergic symptoms are the side effects of the immune system's attack on what is often a harmless noncombatant.

IgE antibodies normally float freely in the blood stream and in the fluid that surrounds the body's tissues. But many also attach to the outside of basophils and similar cells called mast cells. Some immunologists contend that mast cells are nothing more than basophils that have moved outside capillaries and venules to reside in connective tissue. Partially buried in mast cell's membrane, as many as 500,000 IgE antibodies await the arrival of allergens. Contact with an allergen bridges adjacent IgE antibodies, each binding to the offender at a different site, and changes the alignment of the antibodies on the

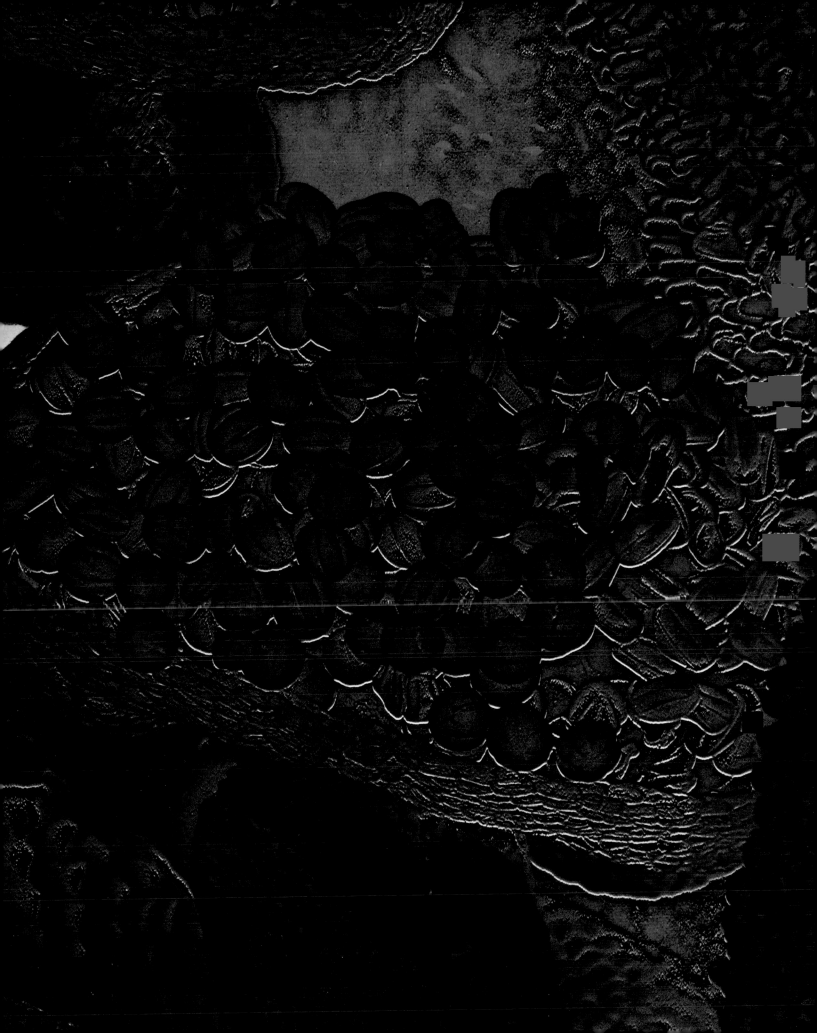

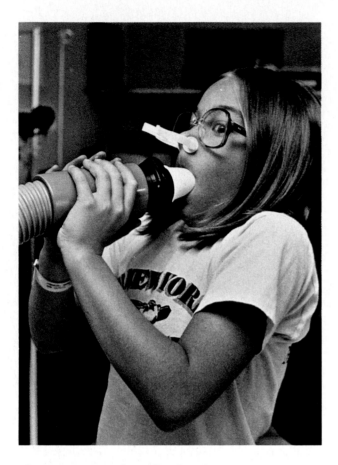

A young patient takes a deep breath and exhales as hard as she can into a spirometer. The device measures the volume of air she expels in one second. A sharp drop in the volume signals the onset of an asthma attack.

surface of the mast cell. The change explodes the mast cell, which dumps histamine, enzymes, chemotactic factors and other substances into the surrounding fluid. Devouring reagin-allergen complexes is an eosinophil's specialty. The body's response is much like an immune response to a virus or bacteria: dilated capillaries, swelling, warmth, redness and sometimes pain. Hay fever is a term coined by nineteenth-century British physician John Bostock, who described its general symptoms:

> About the beginning or middle of June in every year . . . a sensation of heat and fullness is experienced in the eyes. . . . This state gradually increases, until the sensation becomes converted into what may be characterized as a combination of the most acute itching and smarting. . . . A general fullness is experienced in the head, and particularly about the fore part; to this succeeds irritation of the nose, producing sneezing, which occurs in fits of extreme violence, coming on at uncertain intervals. . . . To these local symptoms, are at length added a degree of general indisposition, a great degree of languor, and incapacity for muscular exertion, loss of appetite, emaciation, restless nights, often attended with profuse perspirations, the extremities, however, being generally cold.

Allergies are nothing to sneeze at. Allergic reactions can be debilitating. Americans pay over one billion dollars a year for doctors' visits, drugs and other medical treatment. People who are unable to work because of allergies lose another one billion dollars a year in wages.

Between 2,000 and 4,000 people die of asthma every year. Luckily, allergies can be detected, combatted and often controlled. A skin test, scratching the skin with an allergen-coated needle, will usually prompt a mild reaction in thirty minutes if the individual is allergic. Once the cause of an allergic reaction is found, the most common treatment is to avoid it. Since pollen and some other allergens are so ubiquitous, however, physicians generally prescribe antihistamines to control some of the most uncomfortable symptoms of allergies.

Desensitization, the regular injection of small quantities of allergens, can help immunize some sufferers against their allergies. Steady exposure builds up high quantities of IgG antibodies in the blood stream, in essence creating competition between two classes of antibodies for the same antigen. Allergens that bind to IgG antibodies do not reach the thicket of IgE antibodies coating mast cells. Without the interaction of IgE antibodies, allergens and mast cells, smaller doses of histamine find their way into the body and make the allergic response less potent.

Like other B cells, the cells that produce the IgE antibody probably require the assistance of T cells to churn out effective numbers. Some scientists suspect that allergies are a breakdown in the functioning of helper and suppressor T cells, and that the immune system is mass-producing too much IgE. If this notion proves true, the ability to intervene in the workings of T cells may be the key to controlling allergies.

Some allergens, like poison ivy, elicit a response only from T cells. Since T cells are usually slower to respond to antigens, a reaction to poison ivy might not appear for hours or days after exposure to the allergen. The allergen itself does little or no damage. Poison ivy's itching and blisters are the handiwork of sensitized T cells and their potent lymphokines.

Roughly seven out of ten Americans share a sensitivity to urushiol, the active substance in poison ivy. The urushiol molecule is too small to prompt an immune response of its own. When it creeps through the skin, it joins with other substances, often the body's own proteins. T cells will then attack the large, combined antigen, responding to the molecular configuration of both the carrier protein and the tiny antigen. After the initial immune response, with its creation of antibodies and memory cells, the appearance of the small antigen alone, called a hapten, is enough to provoke a defensive reaction.

In some cases the immune system's reaction to allergens does not stop with localized swelling and tender skin. For some extremely hypersensitive people, exposure to an allergen can cause abdominal pains, fainting and other signs of anaphylactic shock. In someone highly allergic to bee venom, a bee sting can prompt a widespread reaction that dumps massive amounts of hista-

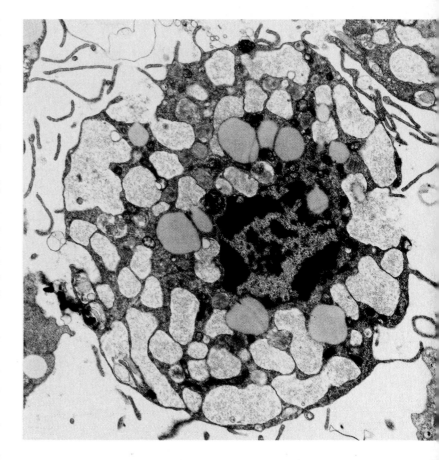

Mast cells cling to the outside of blood vessels and lie just beneath the skin throughout the body. In allergic reactions, the interaction of allergens, antibodies, and mast cells causes the cells to rupture. They dump histamine and other chemicals into surrounding fluid. The mast cell's chemical contents cause the most common allergic symptoms.

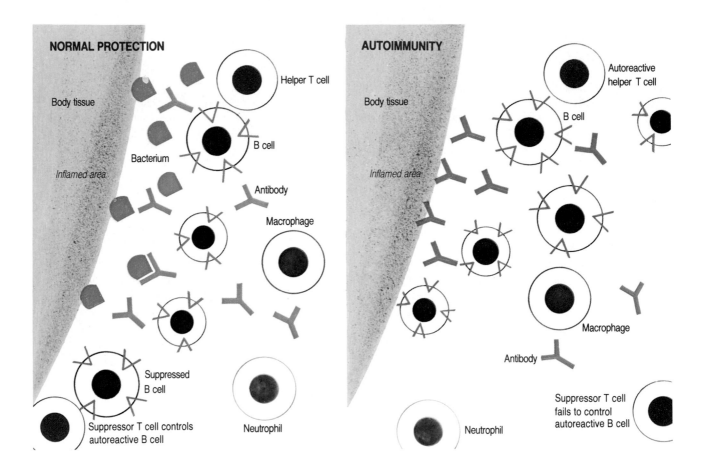

The healthy immune system attacks only invading antigens, left. B cells and helper T cells work together to synthesize antibodies against the invaders. The linking of antigen and antibody calls in neutrophils and macrophages to devour the aliens. Autoreactive B cells, programmed to attack the body's own tissues, are kept under control by suppressor T cells. In an autoimmune response, right, the body's defenders turn traitorous. Suppressor T cells fail to control autoreactive B and helper T cells. The renegade lymphocytes conspire to produce antibodies that bind to healthy tissue. Macrophages and neutrophils, misled by renegade antibodies, attack the body's own cells.

mine into the circulation. Histamine's dilation of small blood vessels and their increased permeability can drain plasma from the vessels into the tissues, producing potentially fatal low blood pressure. Another product of exploding mast cells, called slow-reacting substance of anaphylaxis, or SRS-A, constricts air passages in the lungs, sometimes severely enough to cause suffocation. Although a desensitization serum made from bee venom has become available in the last three years, roughly fifty Americans die every year of insect stings.

Allergies serve no obvious purpose, and that is their great enigma. Seemingly harmless substances prompt annoying and even fatal reactions in some people. A few people seem to be allergic to an incredible variety of ordinary and exotic foods, fibers and chemicals. They must be protected from a host of potential allergens, because their immunological defenses are too eager to destroy "nonself."

Warring With the Self

Like its interactions with the outside world, the immune system's internal checks and balances can go awry, resulting in an autoimmune response, a disorder in which the body attacks itself. One modern theory of immunology, clonal selection, suggests that the pool of stem cells producing lymphocytes to combat disease also produces forbidden clones — lymphocytes targeted against the body's own cells. These renegade lymphocytes treat the body as alien and, unchecked, begin the war of self against self.

During fetal development and the first few months of life, scientists believe, most of these traitorous B and T cells are paralyzed at a crucial stage in development. Proteins and sugars marking the body's cells circulate in the blood stream. These "self-antigens," the theory holds, bind to renegade lymphocytes early in their development, crippling rather than activating the B or T cells. Lymphocytes in the fetus and newborn seem especially susceptible to clonal selection. In experiments with mice, scientists have injected spleen cells from a donor mouse into the thymus of a newborn mouse. The meeting with foreign cells arrests the development of some immature

T cells, preventing the mouse from later rejecting a skin graft from the donor. The procedure fools the mouse's immune system, causing it to regard the foreign tissue as self. More support for the clonal selection theory lies in the fact that proteins from the lens of the eye, which do not encounter lymphocytes during fetal development, prompt an immune response if they are released into the blood stream later in life. The immune system fails to recognize the lens proteins as the body's own, and attacks them.

Since the bone marrow produces about 200,000 lymphocytes per second, some of which assume forbidden identities through the random mistakes of cell division and reproduction, the immune system must protect itself from renegade lymphocytes through life.

The immune system responds most effectively to a certain amount of an antigen in the blood stream and body fluids, what might be called the antigen's optimal dose. The dose varies with every antigen. The presence of an antigen in much smaller or larger amounts induces tolerance rather than immunity. Low doses of antigen maintained in the blood stream over long periods of time can prompt what immunologists call low-zone tolerance. Immature helper T cells targeted for the antigen might respond poorly to a low dose, scientists think. They fail to divide into memory cells and active helper cells and thus do not stimulate the appropriate clone of B cells.

Suppressor T cells play the vital role in preserving low-zone tolerance. While helper T cells perform best after a macrophage presents them with a concentrated dose of antigen, suppressor T cells seem to respond to antigens directly. The injection of low doses of antigens in the blood stream, which normally carries no macrophages, triggers a higher proportion of suppressors to respond than an injection under the skin, where macrophages can ingest the antigen and present it to helper T cells. Stray proteins, bits of cell membranes and nuclei tumbling through the body could trigger renegade helper T and B cells to produce antibodies against the tissues from which the cellular debris came. But as long as a sufficient number of suppressor T cells responds to the same antigens, self-tolerance is preserved.

Activated suppressors recognize and intercept B and T cells. Researchers believe suppressors secrete a lymphokine that calls in macrophages to ingest the renegade lymphocytes. With enough helper T cells crippled, even a larger dose of the antigen introduced later on does not prompt an immune response.

A flood of antigen can create high-zone tolerance, overwhelming even mature B and T cells already sensitized to the antigen. From then on, immunologists believe, the lymphocytes are either temporarily or permanently tolerant, even if they encounter the antigen again. Bone marrow might produce B cells programmed to attack one of the body's own antibodies, which are nothing more than proteins themselves. Small quantities of the antibody in the blood stream might prompt a few of the renegade B cells to mature into plasma cells and memory cells, with the assistance of helper T cells. But huge amounts of the antibody could flood the blood stream quickly, in response to an infection, and the massive dose would overwhelm the helper T and B cells before they could turn against the antibodies.

A lapse in low or high doses allows newly created lymphocytes in the bone marrow to escape paralysis, mature and respond to an optimal dose of an antigen. But as long as low or high doses of an antigen continue to deactivate lymphocytes and suppressors keep a constant watch, the immune system tolerates the antigen. When the antigen in question is one of the body's own proteins, tolerance keeps the immune system from attacking its host.

In all autoimmune responses, self-tolerance breaks down. Drugs or serious infections that destroy suppressor T cells can leave the body vulnerable to an autoimmune response. In some congenital diseases, T cells can be defective. And with age, the number of suppressor T cells in blood and lymph seems to decline, increasing the chance of autoimmune reactions in older people. The failure of suppressor T cells to perform their role, for whatever reasons, may be the key defect in autoimmune disease. The body's immune reaction to itself parallels its response to invading antigens. Not all antigen-antibody complexes formed against the body's own tissues produce the same symptoms. Some, however, open the door to a full-scale attack, involving complement, histamine, chemotaxis, swelling, clotting, agglutination and phagocytosis.

The Body Battles Cancer

Along with preserving tolerance to the body's own tissues, the immune system may oversee an unknown number of other changes and processes in the body. T cells and macrophages have been implicated in controlling cancerous tumors. Like all other cells, cancerous cells present proteins on their cell membranes — markers that identify them as friend or foe. The mutations that occur in the formation of tumors often change the cell's protein markers, labeling it an alien and calling in T cells and macrophages. Indeed, as one scientist puts it, everyone may get cancer once a day, but the immune system tirelessly searches out the malignant cells and destroys them. With age, the influence of the thymus gland wanes and the incidence of cancer increases.

Since the immune system as a whole not only protects the body from invading and cancerous cells, but also disposes of damaged red blood cells and other injured and aging tissues, it is an unflagging monitor of growth and health. As the thymus ages and the dose of thymic hormones in the blood stream declines, the intricate system of cell divisions and hormonal messages that produce potent T cells may crumble too. Many immunologists argue that the winding down of the thymic clock on a genetically inherited timetable may be an integral part of aging itself. A sluggish immune system, creating fewer new T cells, loses some of its power to help, suppress and kill. Without vital T cells to interact with B cells and macrophages, the body may be unable to protect itself from both hostile bacteria and the perpetual cellular mistakes and mutations that inevitably accompany life.

Its link with aging only underscores the immune system's heavy responsibilities for preserving identity and life. It is an invisible multitude of cells, proteins and chemicals that marks the boundary between self and nonself, health and disease, growth and decline — a mobilized army warring in life's defense.

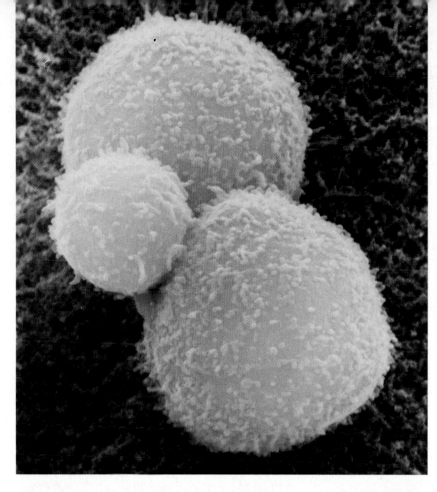

Killer T cells are one of the body's defenses against cancer. Magnified 9,000 times, a small killer T cell assaults two larger cancer cells, top. As a killer T cell destroys a cancer cell, bottom, blisters appear on the dying cell's membrane. The two photomicrographs by Andrejs Liepins of Memorial University of Newfoundland in Canada illustrate one of the immune system's most important functions — surveillance. Life and health depend on its sleepless watch for enemies both within and without.

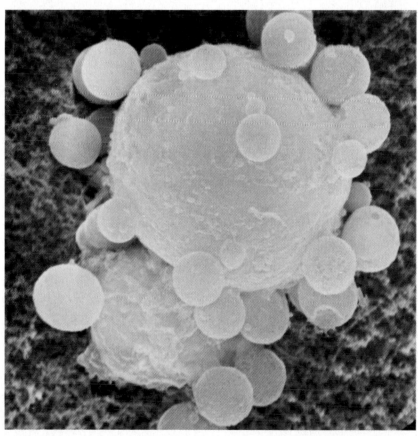

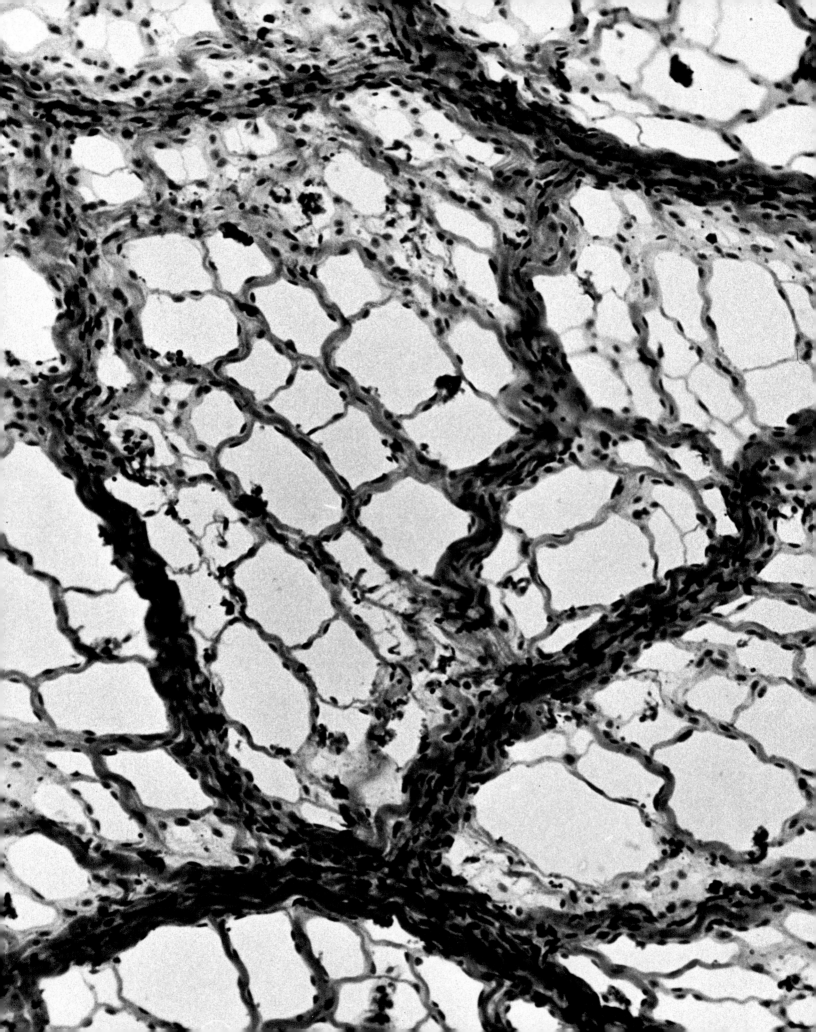

Chapter 6

Perils of the River

Like rivers branching into streams, arteries channel blood into tiny arterioles. White-water canoeists know well how calm streams can turn to violent rapids without warning. So, too, can blood, the river of life, pose sudden perils.

Every February on the Mediterranean island of Sardinia, children suddenly become languid. They lose interest in school work, complain of dizziness and fall asleep in class. Adults exhibit similar behavior. But it is not spring fever that for centuries has afflicted as much as 35 percent of the island's population. Some even die from the perennial sickness.

Intrigued by the mysterious disorder, Marcello Siniscalco of Memorial Sloan-Kettering Cancer Center in New York and Arno G. Motulsky of the University of Washington traveled to the mountainous island in 1959. Testing the population's blood samples, they found abnormal red blood cells in those who were sick. The tests revealed that nearly all who suffered lacked the gene responsible for the production of glucose-6-phosphate dehydrogenase, an enzyme important in the formation of normal red blood cells.

They diagnosed hemolytic anemia, a genetic disorder in which red blood cells periodically become abnormally fragile and die. Although the precise mechanism is unknown, scientists believe that when triggered by a variety of substances, including certain drugs and vegetable toxins, the abnormal cells burst, releasing oxygen-carrying hemoglobin pigments into the blood stream. This can cause the lethargic feeling associated with all anemias, as well as abdominal pains and more serious problems, as impurities from dead red blood cells accumulate.

The scientists next set out to find the substance among the rolling grasslands and ancient cork forests that provoked the springtime sickness. Scouring the island, they found the fava bean, a native plant that flowers during spring. It is a plant that, Siniscalco observed, "has had a bad reputation ever since 500 B.C. when the Greek philosopher Pythagoras barred his followers from eating it or even from walking through fields in which it was growing." It was becoming

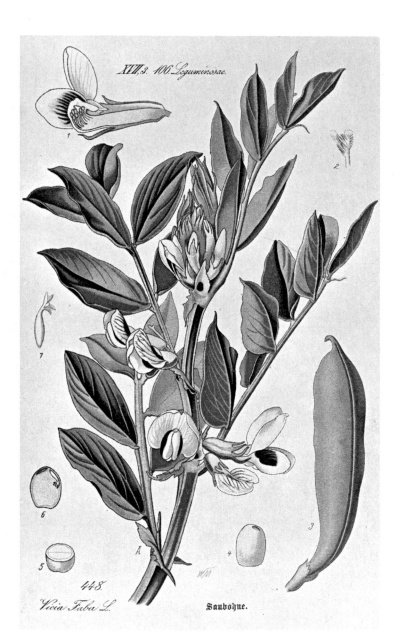

XVII,3. 106.Leguminosae.

448.
Vicia Faba L.   Saubohne.

clear that only those with the defective gene who had eaten raw or partly-cooked fava beans or inhaled pollen from its flower experienced attacks.

Within two years, Motulsky developed a simple blood test that could determine if the enzyme was absent and thus provide a genetic marker for those susceptible to the disease. The scientists began to screen Sardinians for the marker, warning those who were predisposed to the disease to avoid fava beans during the flowering season. Soon, spring-feverlike behavior and the debilitating symptoms of the anemia declined.

Predicting Disease

Testing blood for genetic markers may someday enable doctors to predict the likelihood of a patient's contracting a wide range of diseases later in life. Stanford University scientists have designed blood-testing techniques that one member of the group, Edgar Engleman, calls "absolutely revolutionary." These tests would predict whether a person might suffer future illnesses such as diabetes, peptic ulcer, malaria or heart disease. At the California Institute of Technology, investigators have devised a computerized blood test for analyzing chromosomes, strands of organic material which carry genes. The test would provide concise descriptions of suspected genetic abnormalities and predict the likelihood of disease. Some experts believe that within twenty years, computers will analyze blood samples for genetic markers to determine an individual's risk of contracting more than 100 illnesses. A computer printout would list foods, drugs and geographical locations that might act as catalysts for disease.

Other researchers are analyzing blood for hormones thought to be secreted by some cancers. The hormones could prove to be markers for certain thyroid, lung and gastrointestinal cancers even before tumors appear. Although the clinical value of this test has not been determined, researchers hope it will enable them to diagnose cancers at an early stage when they are most responsive to treatment.

Another blood test that holds promise for early diagnosis of cancer is being developed by researchers at Canada's McGill University. The scientists found that cancerous cells, unlike normal white blood cells, do not adhere to glass surfaces when incubated. Their new blood assay would detect this identifying trait, which seems most pronounced during early development of disease. Researchers at Pennsylvania State University have devised a single test to screen blood for nearly all known cancers. This method, which would greatly simplify diagnoses now requiring more than a dozen tests for specific cancers, measures levels of protein and carbohydrate compounds called glycoproteins in the blood stream. Certain glycoproteins are secreted only by cancer cells. If this technique gains approval from the U.S. Food and Drug Administration, it could become a routine part of physical examinations.

Scientists at Bell Telephone Laboratories are working on a simpler, more accurate test to measure levels of bilirubin, a bile pigment, in the blood of unborn babies. Ten percent of all babies are thought to have excessive levels of bilirubin. If this substance accumulates in the blood, it causes jaundice or irreversible brain damage. The five-minute test, requiring only three drops of fetal blood, isolates the wavelength of light bilirubin emits when exposed to blue light. It also determines how much more of the potentially toxic substance the baby's blood stream can safely hold. Should the test show the infant's blood to be saturated with bilirubin, doctors could take lifesaving steps immediately after delivery. This technique is also used to detect high levels of lead in the blood, a sign of lead poisoning.

A Sweet-Tasting Poison

Small children are the primary victims of lead poisoning. So toxic is lead that only three small chips of lead-based paint eaten every week for several months will cause serious harm. Once consumed, the sweet-tasting metal is absorbed into the blood and bones. Lead can be excreted only in small quantities. Excessive amounts poison the blood, causing abdominal cramps and lethargy and, in severe cases, brain damage and coma. A child with abnormally high levels of lead in his blood must be kept away from it long enough for his system to excrete the overload. It takes twice as long to remove lead from the blood stream as it takes to accumulate it.

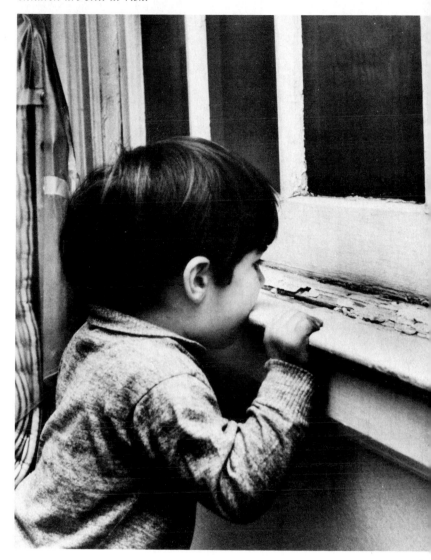

A child need eat only three small chips of lead-based paint each week for several months to suffer serious lead-poisoning problems. Health officials estimate that 100,000 children are still at risk.

In severe anemia, red blood cells deficient in hemoglobin appear bell-shaped, but flatten out when smeared across a slide for study, below. Up to 20 percent of all American women have anemia.

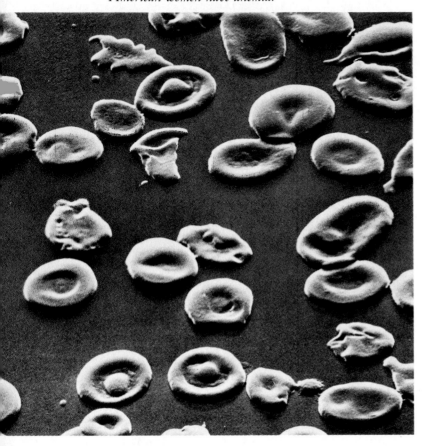

Thirty years ago, paint manufacturers stopped putting lead into interior paint. But researchers at the Centers for Disease Control in Atlanta estimate that of the fifteen million children under six years old in the United States, 100,000 are still at risk, exposed to old paint.

Clair C. Patterson and Dorothy Settle of the Division of Geological and Planetary Sciences at the California Institute of Technology believe children are not the only ones threatened by lead poisoning. The geochemists claim that for decades researchers failed to correctly identify lead contamination levels in processed foods sold in cans with lead-soldered seams. Patterson and Settle think current definitions of classic lead poisoning are inadequate.

Lead poisoning may not be only a modern dilemma. Sociologist Seabury Gilfillan believes lead poisoning might have contributed to the fall of the Roman Empire. Water pipes in the Roman aqueduct system were made of lead, as were cups, bowls, cosmetics and certain medicines. Romans used lead-lined pots to boil grape juice into a syrup for sweetening their wine. Once their blood was contaminated by enormous amounts of lead, many aristocrats, Gilfillan thinks, became sterile. Miscarriages and still-births were common. Gilfillan cites the Roman aristocracy's "high death rates as well as its low birth rate" to support the theory. Two research teams have tested bones believed to be those of ancient Romans. Both found high levels of lead compared with those found in other bone samples from the same period. But it is not certain if the lead deposits resulted from poisoning or from absorption of lead from soil after burial.

The "Green Sickness"

Anemia nearly always accompanies lead poisoning. Caused by a decrease in red blood cells, or in their hemoglobin content, anemia can be much more serious than "tired blood." It can result from nutritional deficiencies, bleeding or a disease of the bone marrow, where red blood cells are produced. Anemia often accompanies liver or thyroid disease, rheumatoid arthritis and internal infection. In mild cases, the disease might produce only a lack of energy. Pallor, particularly in the palms of the hands, the fingernails and the lining of the eyelids, is often a sign of anemia. In severe cases, its symptoms include headache, ringing in the ears, vertigo, irritability, shortness of breath and rapid pulse. In advanced stages, menstruation ceases and libido wanes.

Because severe iron deficiency anemia sometimes causes a pallor with a greenish tint, anemia was once called the "green sickness," or chlorosis. In the seventeenth century, women with chlorosis were said to have the "virgin's disease" because Europeans then equated pallor with sexual innocence. After experimenting with a variety of treatments, physicians in 1681 began prescribing preparations of iron rust or filings boiled in wine. Although these remedies were often successful, not until 1832 was there conclusive proof linking iron deficiency with anemia.

At least one-fifth of the world's population suffers from iron deficiency anemia, according to

CAUSES OF ANEMIA

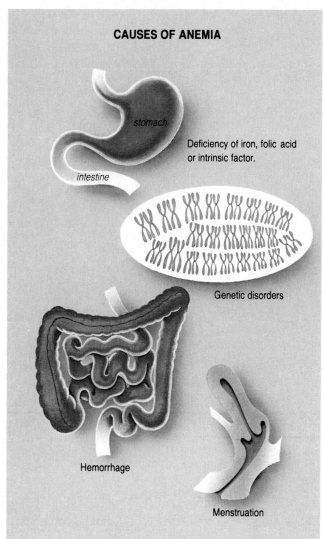

stomach

Deficiency of iron, folic acid
or intrinsic factor.

intestine

Genetic disorders

Hemorrhage

Menstruation

CONSEQUENCES OF ANEMIA

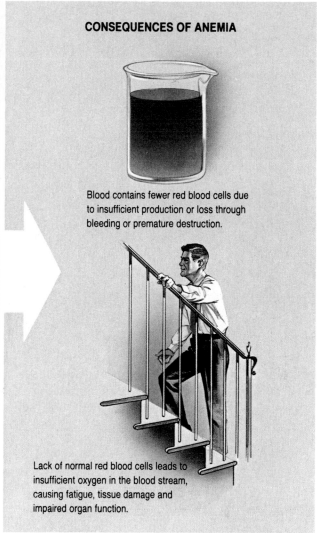

Blood contains fewer red blood cells due
to insufficient production or loss through
bleeding or premature destruction.

Lack of normal red blood cells leads to
insufficient oxygen in the blood stream,
causing fatigue, tissue damage and
impaired organ function.

the World Health Organization. The most common cause in adults is blood loss from menstruation or intestinal bleeding, but in children it is usually attributed to a diet low in iron. In the United States, as many as 20 percent of all women of child-bearing age and 33 percent of all children under six suffer from this anemia. The elderly are also vulnerable.

Iron deficiency anemia among young men might not be as rare as previously believed. Yale University investigators recently found an increased incidence of the illness among adolescent boys. A study by British researchers found the disease in many male army recruits.

Vitamin deficiencies can also produce anemia. Lack of folic acid, one of the B vitamins, is the most common vitamin deficiency anemia. It is found among heavy drinkers, patients receiving antiepileptic medication and women taking oral contraceptives. Like alcohol, these medications

Caused by a decrease in the number of red blood cells, anemia can result from a wide range of conditions including chronic bleeding, diseases of the bone marrow, inability to absorb vitamin B-12 and deficiency of iron in the diet. With fewer red cells circulating in the blood stream, less oxygen is available to the brain and other organs and tissues that require oxygen to carry out normal functions. Pernicious anemia, one of the most severe forms, can be fatal.

Flowing freely through blood vessels, healthy red blood cells, right, deliver oxygen and other nutrients throughout the body. During a sickle cell crisis, red cells gel into crescentlike shapes and clog blood vessels, below. Pain develops as tissues and organs starve for oxygen. The crisis ends when enough cells are able to squeeze through congested vessels to the lungs, where oxygen restores them to normal.

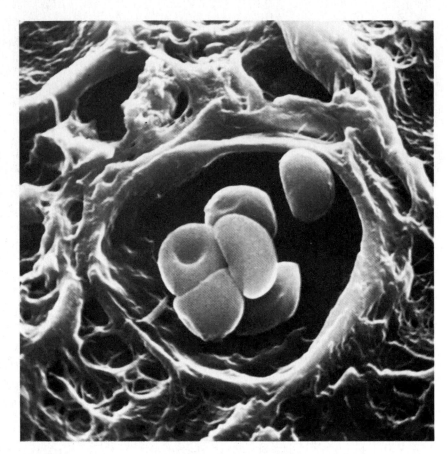

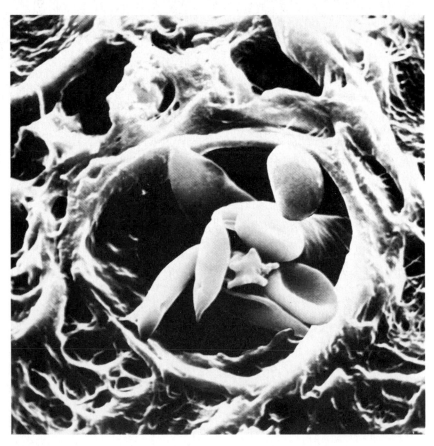

interfere with the body's utilization of folic acid. A deficiency of vitamin B-12 can eventually lead to pernicious anemia, a severe anemia characterized by abnormally large red blood cells, spinal cord lesions and gastrointestinal disorders. The condition is caused by lack of what doctors call the intrinsic factor, a substance that enables the intestines to absorb the vitamin B complex. Unless treated with B-12 shots, this anemia can lead to disorders of the nervous system and death.

An Ancient Mutation

Perhaps no anemia is as debilitating and unpredictable as sickle cell, a genetic disease which afflicts one in every 600 American blacks. Some patients suffer painful attacks — sickling crises — from childhood on, while others mysteriously do not experience them until middle age.

A severe crisis begins when abnormal proteins cause surrounding red cells to gel into sicklelike shapes. The victim first senses pain when sickled cells begin to clog veins and arteries. As fewer and fewer red blood cells pass through congested blood vessels, tissues and joints become starved for oxygen and other nutrients. Intestinal cramps often follow. The crisis ends when enough sickled cells are able to squeeze through blood vessels to the lungs, where they obtain sufficient oxygen to restore them to a normal state.

A severe crisis can occur in any part of the body and can vary in intensity from one victim to the next. Sickling that clogs vessels in the hand might simply cause swelling and discomfort. Attacks occurring near a vital organ are much more serious and painful because they disrupt the organ's functions. Over time, severe crises can destroy the spleen, kidneys and other organs. Sickle cell victims are especially vulnerable to viruses and other infections as the disease weakens natural defenses. Children face an added risk because crises during childhood can lead to seizure or stroke.

Yuet Wai Kan and Andree M. Dozy of the University of California at San Francisco have traced two forms of sickle cell anemia back thousands of years to various parts of Africa. According to their theory, the disease began when the genes of at least two Africans underwent a

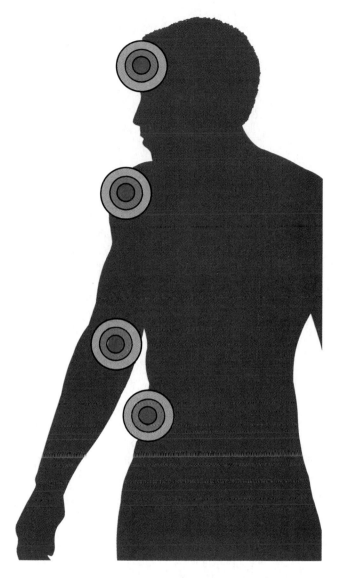

Sickle cell crises are unpredictable, varying in frequency and intensity from one person to the next. A crisis can occur anywhere in the body. Most often, sickled cells clog vessels in the joints, causing excruciating pain. Severe crises can eventually destroy vital organs. Because a child's blood vessels are not fully developed, children who suffer from sickle cell anemia have a greater chance of seizure or stroke than adult sufferers.

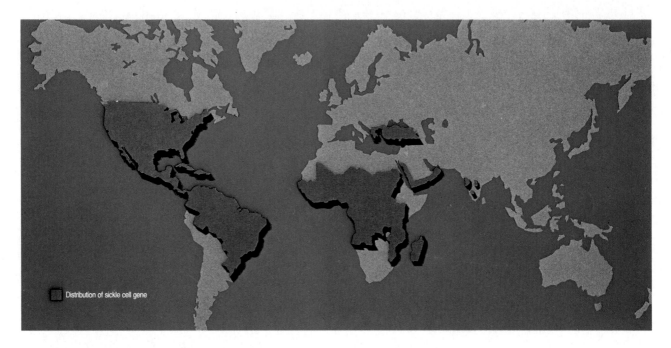

Distribution of sickle cell gene

change or mutation that caused cells to sickle. When these genetic changes occurred, malaria was ravaging the continent. Those with the mutant gene were more resistant to the disease. While thousands of Africans died from malaria, those harboring the sickle cell gene survived, passing the mutation to offspring. Rockefeller University parasitologist Milton J. Friedman suggests sickle cell carriers survived because the malarial parasites that had infected their red cells had starved from lack of oxygen.

Studying blood samples from sickle cell sufferers throughout the world, Kan and Dozy traced the form of the disease that afflicts blacks in the United States to a small area in west Africa. Yet, the genetic disorder does not affect only blacks. The researchers have gathered evidence showing that the form of sickle cell anemia found among Turks, Sicilians and other Mediterranean people evolved from a larger region encompassing east Africa, India and Saudi Arabia.

Many more people possess a single defective gene, called the sickle cell trait, than actually have the disease. The single trait is not the disease and carries none of the dangers of sickle cell anemia. But two healthy individuals, each carrying the defective gene, have a one-in-four chance

of together passing the genes, and thus the disease, to their offspring. A recipient of the double trait will have the disease. To show that carriers of the trait do not suffer as a result of the single defect, researchers made a study of 579 black athletes in the National Football League in 1973. The single trait surfaced in thirty-nine players.

New research shows that the causes of sickle cell may not be purely genetic. University of Kansas scientists found that membrane proteins surrounding red blood cells were abnormal in both quantity and quality among sickle cell patients who had moderate or severe symptoms. Those with the most severe symptoms had the greatest abnormalities. Scientists now seek ways to alter the abnormal proteins in the severely afflicted as a means of relieving pain. The only current treatments for sickle cell anemia are vaccinations for common infections, pain medication and oxygen administered during crises. Reducing sodium levels in the blood and increasing fluid intake appear to decrease the frequency and intensity of sickling crises in some patients.

Experimental treatments offer some hope. Because sickled cells become normal when hemoglobin S molecules come into contact with oxygen, sodium cyanate, which helps cells retain

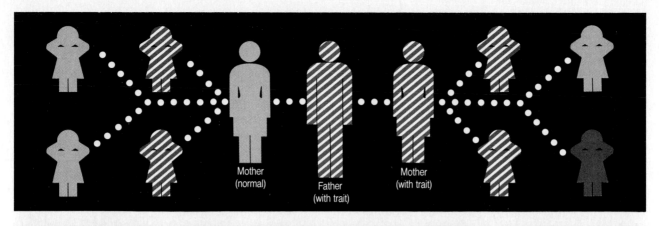

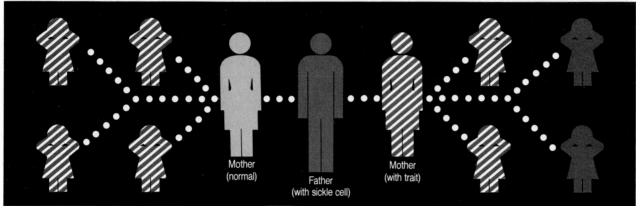

oxygen, sometimes brings relief. But its side effects can be dangerous. Albert L. Babb, a biomedical engineer, and Belding Scribner, professor of medicine at the University of Washington, have begun testing an advanced version of a kidney dialysis machine for treating sickle cell patients. Dialysis is a method used for filtering and cleansing blood of certain components. The sickle cell patient's blood would be slowly drawn from his body into a "reaction vessel" where sodium cyanate would be added. The sodium cyanate would then be removed and the treated blood returned to the patient's body. A computer would monitor blood chemistry during treatment and automatically turn the machine off if sodium cyanate levels were to become toxic.

Erythrocytosis, another serious blood disease, is the opposite of anemia. In this disorder, red blood cell levels are excessively high. Blood vessels, clogged with red cells, cannot funnel enough oxygen and other nutrients to the bone marrow. The starving marrow begins producing greater amounts of red cells. As the cycle progresses, blood becomes so thick with red cells that clots form, threatening stroke or heart attack.

A common treatment for erythrocytosis is venesection, a method somewhat reminiscent of

The map on the opposite page shows the geographical distribution of the mutant sickle cell gene. Some scientists believe the disease began in Africa during a malaria epidemic, then spread to the Mediterranean region and the western hemisphere. The illustration, above, shows how the mutation is passed from one generation to the next.

bloodletting. Instead of using leeches and cupping glasses, however, doctors draw seven to ten ounces of blood through a needle placed in the vein of a patient's arm. The lost blood is replaced with plasma, which temporarily reduces red blood cell count to normal levels. Most patients also take drugs that help thin the blood. Doctors sometimes give injections of radioactive phosphorus. Carried to the bones, this chemical stops bone marrow from producing excess red cells.

The "Kissing" Disease

In another blood disorder, infectious mononucleosis, patients have elevated levels of leukocytes, white blood cells. Striking mostly between the ages of seventeen and thirty, mononucleosis was nicknamed the "kissing disease" in the 1950s by Robert Hoagland, then chief physician at West Point Military Academy. Hoagland coined the term after noticing an alarming increase in the incidence of the disease among cadets returning to West Point from Christmas vacation. Medical casebooks also report epidemics of mononucleosis among sailors five or six weeks after returning from shore leave. The disease can also be spread by common use of eating and drinking utensils and by blood transfusions from a donor who once had the disease.

Most scientists now believe mononucleosis is caused by a virus. The discovery that led to this theory came about by accident. In 1967, when researchers were studying the Epstein-Barr virus, which caused facial tumors in African children, one of the laboratory technicians contracted mononucleosis. Before her illness, her blood test did not show any Epstein-Barr antibodies. After her bout with the disease, antibodies appeared.

Virtual proof that the Epstein-Barr virus causes mononucleosis came from an eight-year study conducted at Yale University in the 1960s. For years, doctors there had gathered blood samples from freshmen. They found that students whose blood had not contained Epstein-Barr antibodies when they entered Yale, but who later contracted mononucleosis, harbored the antibody. Those whose initial blood tests showed the antibody were apparently immune to the disease. Scientists are still puzzled as to why a virus that

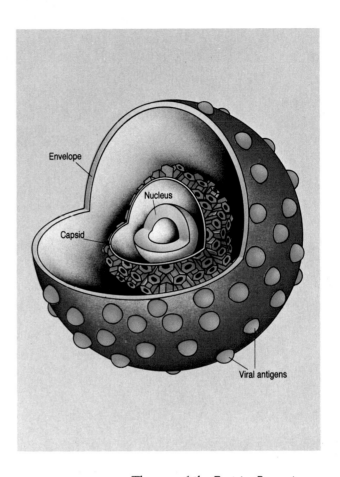

The core of the Epstein-Barr virus, above, is a doughnut-shaped nucleus containing genetic information that propagates the virus throughout the body. Surrounding this is a protein shell, made up of hollow protein components, and a protective envelope studded with antigens. During infection, the envelope fuses with a host cell, forming a gateway for the virus to enter. The invading virus fools the cell's machinery into manufacturing new virus particles.

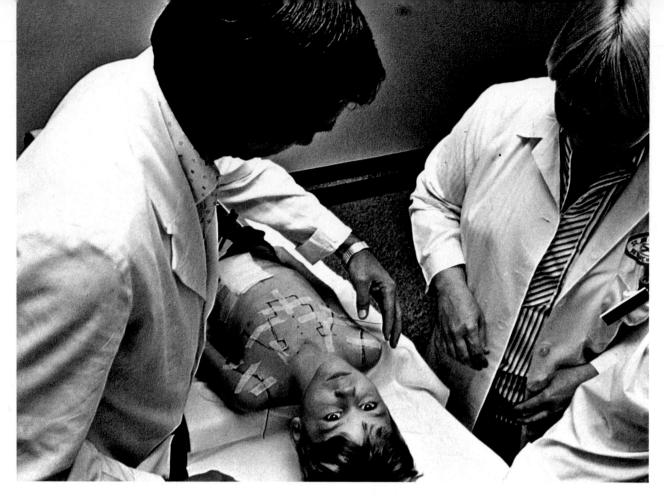

Medical technicians prepare a leuke-mia patient for radiation therapy. "Total therapy," which combines radiation with anticancer drugs, has brought remission of symptoms in many cases.

disfigures children in Africa causes an uncomfortable but brief blood disorder in Americans. Some researchers believe environmental and genetic factors might be involved. Most doctors agree that one attack of mononucleosis guarantees lifelong immunity. Fewer than 1 percent of patients experience complications, although liver and kidney functions must be closely monitored.

Some scientists describe mononucleosis as a self-limited leukemia because patients have high levels of abnormally formed white blood cells, a condition also found in certain blood cancers. In mononucleosis, however, production of these cells is temporary, while in leukemia, cells continue to multiply uncontrollably.

Two common forms of leukemia are acute lymphoblastic leukemia, which affects mostly young children, and acute myeloblastic leukemia, one of the most intractable blood cancers. In both types, abnormal white blood cells are produced in such large amounts that they eventually accumulate within the body's vital organs, impeding their functions and leading to death.

Perhaps the most promising new treatment for leukemia is "total therapy." Developed by scientists at St. Jude Children's Research Hospital in Memphis, Tennessee, it combines anticancer

140

medication with radiation therapy. Given primarily to victims of acute lymphoblastic leukemia, total therapy has brought permanent remission of symptoms in many cases. Approximately half of all leukemic children who have received total therapy remain symptom-free for two-and-a-half years, and 70 to 80 percent of them remain in remission for four years.

Acute myeloblastic leukemia (AML) strikes mostly middle-aged adults. Twenty thousand Americans succumb to it each year. In this disease, abnormal white cells invade bone marrow, preventing the marrow from producing normal white, red and platelet cells.

AML is beginning to respond to a new method of chemotherapy. At the National Institutes of Health's Cancer Research Center in Baltimore, Maryland, patients take a combination of five anticancer drugs until signs of remission appear. Only four of the twenty-two patients who have completed the program have had relapses. About 25 percent of those who have responded have remained "at least four to five years disease-free," according to Acting Associate Director Peter Wiernick. "The important thing," says Howard Weinstein of the Sidney Farber Cancer Research Institute in Boston, "is to tell people there is a reasonable chance today for long survival."

Other AML treatments that appear promising include intensive chemotherapy and "total-body irradiation," in which the entire body is subjected to X-rays, followed by transplants of bone marrow, usually donated by members of the immediate family. Researchers are also attempting to formulate safe antibiotic medications to prevent infections brought on by the body's lowered resistance, caused, in turn, by anticancer drugs and radiation therapy.

Researchers have long been aware that cats can contract leukemia apparently from an infectious virus. Although there is no documented case of a human falling victim to a viral leukemia, one study showed that 64 percent of leukemia patients had either direct or indirect physical contact with leukemia victims before coming down with the disease. Another study conducted in the late 1960s showed "a significant relationship between exposure to sick cats and the subsequent

The large cells stained red, below, are white blood cells as they appear in a blood smear taken from a leukemia patient. In this blood cancer, abnormal white cells multiply relentlessly, clogging vital organs.

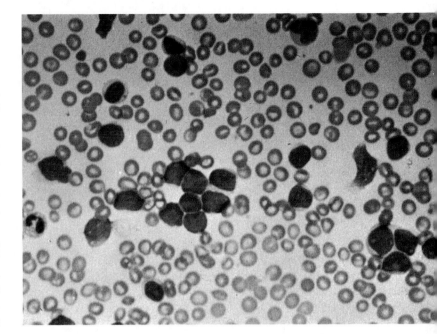

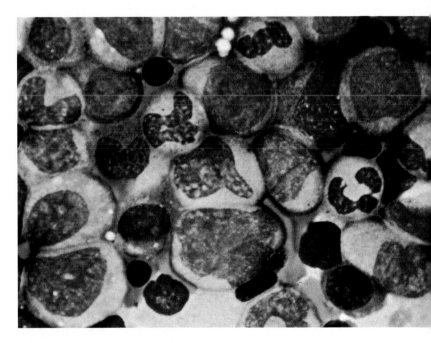

White blood cells have invaded the cavity of this bone marrow sample, above, taken from a leukemia patient. The cavity normally contains immature blood cells, connective tissue, blood vessels and fat cells.

141

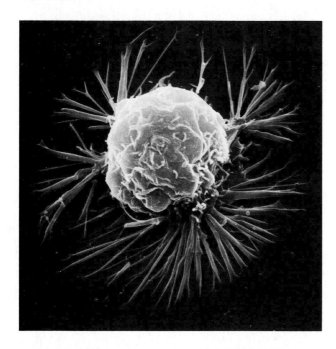

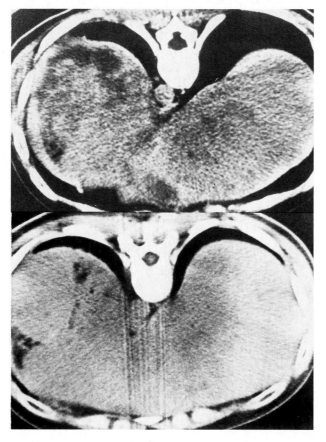

development of leukemia." An eleven-year study by a University of Florida researcher found an unusually high incidence of leukemia among veterinarians who had treated leukemic cats.

Scientists are gathering clues about how viruses might cause cancers in animals. They have observed that viruses in mice somehow exchange genetically-encoded substances with their host and acquire genes that cause leukemia. These "proviruses" may number in the hundreds. But whether this finding is relevant to human leukemias is uncertain.

Fooling the Immune System

Any one of the four million cells that divide each second in a normal adult's body could become malignant. It takes only that single cancerous cell to produce a tumor. At first, the malignancy is only a few millimeters in diameter. Without a network of blood vessels to supply nutrients and remove waste, the cancerous cell remains dormant and relatively harmless for years. How such a cell escapes detection by the body's immune system is one of the most perplexing problems cancer specialists face. Normally, the body's defense system rallies against harmful substances by sending white blood cells to attack invading cells. But cancerous cells somehow avoid this warning system or inhibit immune responses.

Harold and Ann Dvorak at Massachussetts General Hospital and W. Hallowell Churchill at Peter Bent Brigham Hospital in Boston theorize that some malignant cells secrete a gel made of fibrin, a clotting factor in blood. The gel envelops the tumor and fools the immune system into thinking the tumor is actually a healing wound. At the same time, the cancer cells secrete a chemical that stimulates nearby blood vessels to send out capillaries toward the tumor colony. The capillaries eventually penetrate the tumor and provide it with a supply of nutrients and a mechanism for the speedy removal of waste. As the tumor grows, the pathologists theorize, it secretes a substance that diverts immune cells from the expanding cocoon and it begins to dissolve the fibrin shell from the inside, allowing itself more room to grow. Research is under way to develop a substance that would melt away the

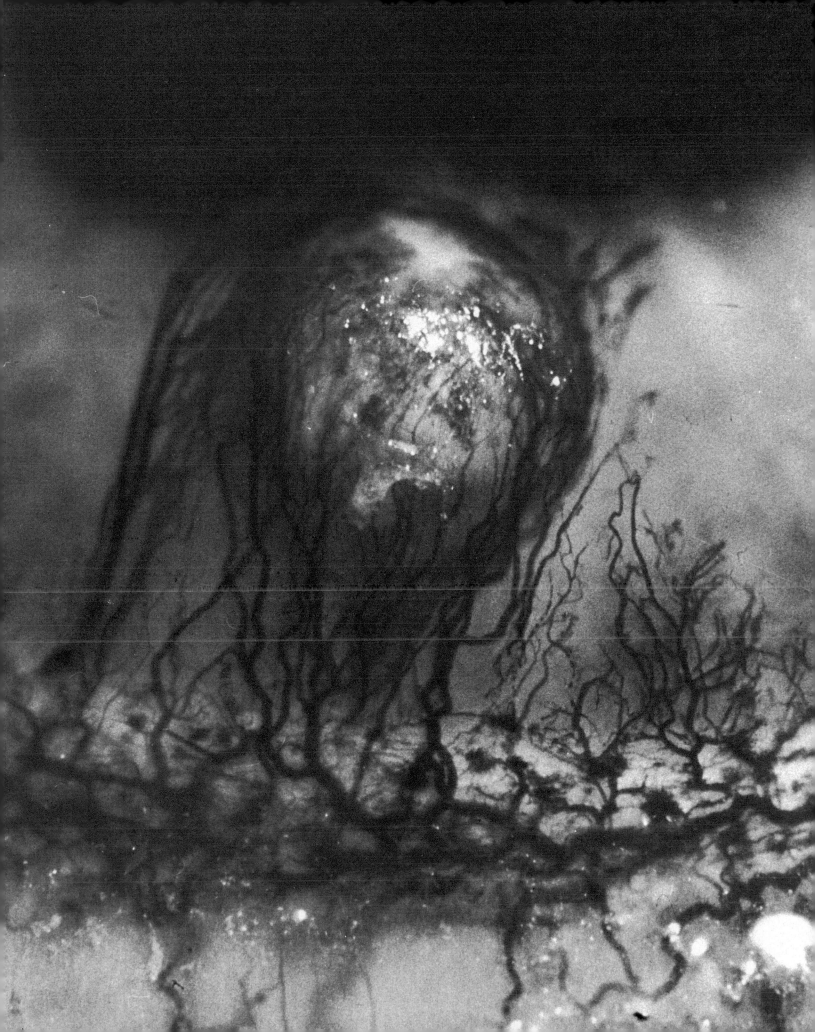

Using gene-splicing techniques, researchers mass-produce interferon, below. First, they cut a ring of genetic material, then place beside it a strand of DNA containing information for production of interferon.

Operating on genes much smaller than a speck of dust, technicians connect the gene possessing blueprints for the production of interferon with the ends of the strand, forming a new genetic ring.

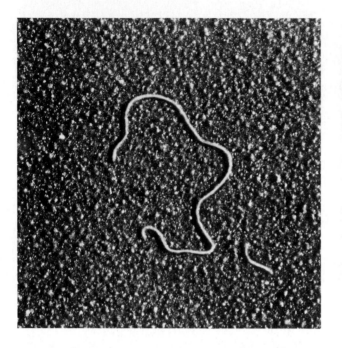

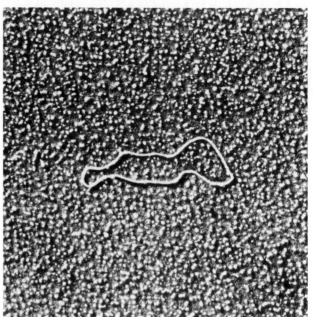

cocoon from the outside and expose the tumor to the full force of the immune system. Other researchers are attempting to develop a chemical that would starve the tumor by inhibiting capillaries from reaching it.

Another approach is immunoglobulin therapy, a radioactive technique making use of a kind of feedback loop linking ferritin, a protein secreted from a cancerous liver tumor, with antibodies from a rabbit's blood. Doctors extract the protein, purify it and inject it into a rabbit. The animal's immune system immediately manufactures antibodies called antiferritin. After removing it from the rabbit's blood, doctors tag this substance with radioactive iodine and inject it into the patient. Antiferritin particles gravitate toward the tumor, releasing a continuous dose of cancer-destroying radiation but leaving normal cells unharmed. To avoid contaminating others, patients undergoing immunoglobulin therapy must live for a week behind a lead wall. While sequestered, they take their own temperatures and measure their pulse rates and intake of liquid. Although immunoglobulin therapy is not considered a cure, it has brought about prolonged remission in patients with liver cancer. The method is now being tested for blood cancers.

Researchers at New York's Memorial Sloan-Kettering Cancer Center recently found proteins isolated from mouse blood that kill cancerous tumors. Saul Green and his coworkers have isolated similar proteins in human blood. These "normal human globulins," the researchers believe, might be vital natural defenses against cancer in both humans and animals.

Interferon is another protein produced naturally within the body. While some researchers have hailed it as an anticancer drug of great promise, others are more cautious. The American Cancer Society believes that initial studies using an impure form of interferon show the drug to be of questionable value. In recent interferon tests the society conducted, "some significant response" was shown in only four of eleven patients with multiple myeloma, a painful bone marrow cancer. The drug proved partially successful in just five of sixteen breast cancer victims.

Yet, in another study, interferon either shrank tumors or stopped them from spreading in 160 of 220 patients. Mathilde Krim, codirector of the interferon laboratory at Sloan-Kettering, feels the drug "opens up a new form of cancer treatment that is nontoxic. There's no nausea, no vomiting, no diarrhea or the other side effects of chemo-

Technicians then insert the new genetic ring into the common and harmless bacteria Escherichia coli, endowing it with the capability of mass-producing interferon for therapeutic use in humans.

The coded bacteria can be grown in vats. Processed under specially controlled laboratory conditions, each gram of Escherichia coli *can be made to yield as many as 10,000 units of interferon.*

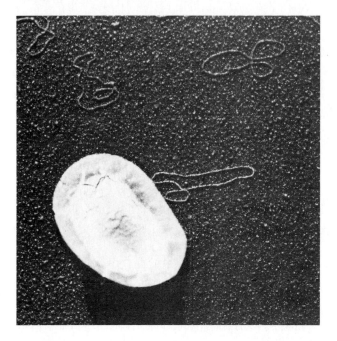

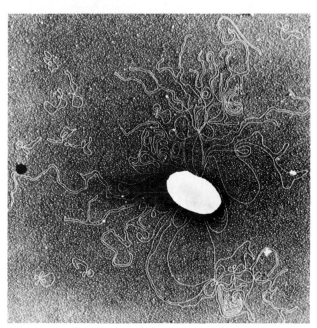

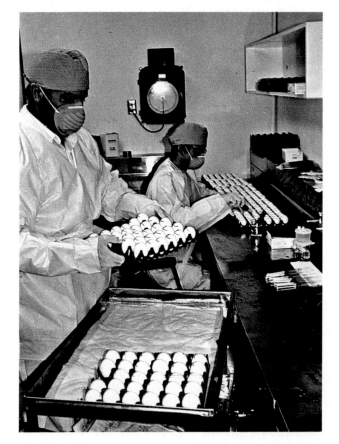

Technicians, left, carry trays of eggs infected with a virus that induces interferon production. When exposed to the virus, cells react by producing interferon. Technicians then add a chemical which separates interferon from the cultured cells.

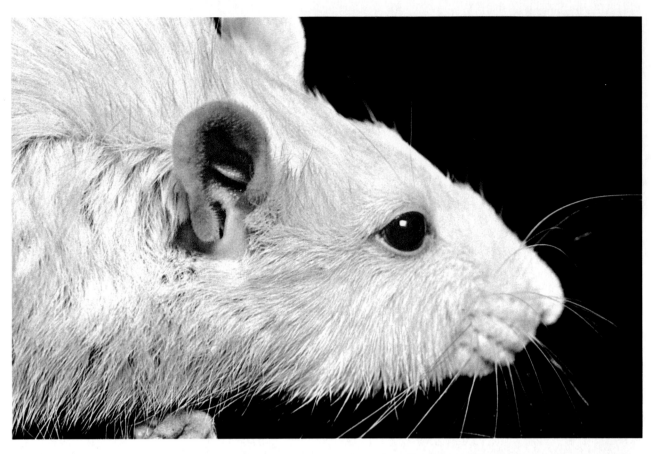

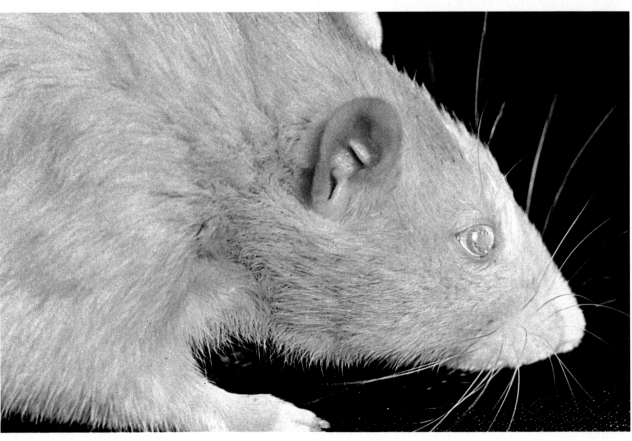

therapy." Krim believes the drug could also prevent viral infection in cancer patients.

Side effects from interferon are just now coming to light. Large doses have killed laboratory
mice. Some humans receiving the drug experience a lethargic condition known as "interferon
malaise." Taken in high doses, interferon also appears to suppress production of bone marrow.

A team of physicians at Stanford University
reports interferon seems to help relieve serum
hepatitis, a viral disease that attacks the liver and
poisons the blood with bile, a mixture of enzymes and other substances that help digest
food. Produced by the liver, bile is normally excreted through the intestines. As the virus infects
the liver, capillaries become blocked and prevent
the removal of bile through normal routes. Bile
spills into the blood stream, and the kidneys, the
blood's filters, cannot remove it quickly enough.

A hepatitis patient complains first of exhaus-
tion and loss of appetite. Next, urine and stools
darken. As the disease progresses and bile accumulates in body tissues, the skin darkens and the
whites of the eyes become yellow. Hepatitis is
fatal in roughly 1 percent of all patients. About
15 percent suffer lasting complications.

There are two types of hepatitis: infectious
hepatitis, which is spread through physical contact, and serum hepatitis, caused chiefly by
transfusions of infected blood. Scientists are not
sure if the two types are caused by two different
viruses or by mutations of the same virus.

As many as 150,000 cases of post-transfusion
hepatitis occur each year in the United States, a
mere fraction of the total number of patients receiving transfusions. In Japan, the probability of
contracting hepatitis after a transfusion is much
greater. To combat the problem, Japanese researchers have developed a petroleum-based
chemical called Fluosol that can be substituted
for human blood during transfusion. Because it is
synthetic, Fluosol carries no risk of hepatitis.

A vaccine against hepatitis was developed during the 1960s. While examining more than
100,000 blood samples from Eskimos, American
Indians, East Asians and Pacific islanders, Baruch
S. Blumberg of the Institute for Cancer Research
in Philadelphia and D. Carlton Gajdusek of the

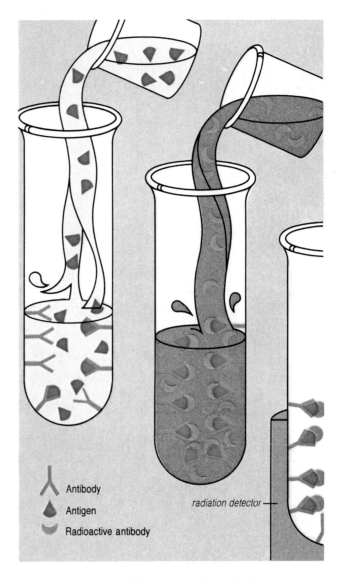

Antibody

Antigen

Radioactive antibody

radiation detector

*Blood is analyzed for hepatitis
through a radioimmunoassay test,
above. A patient's blood serum is
added to a test tube lined with
hepatitis antibodies. Hepatitis antigens present in the sample link with
the antibodies. The patient's serum
is removed and radioactive hepatitis
antibodies, which adhere to the antigen, are added. Now two antibodies
sandwich the antigen. The presence
of hepatitis antigens is determined
by measuring radioactivity.*

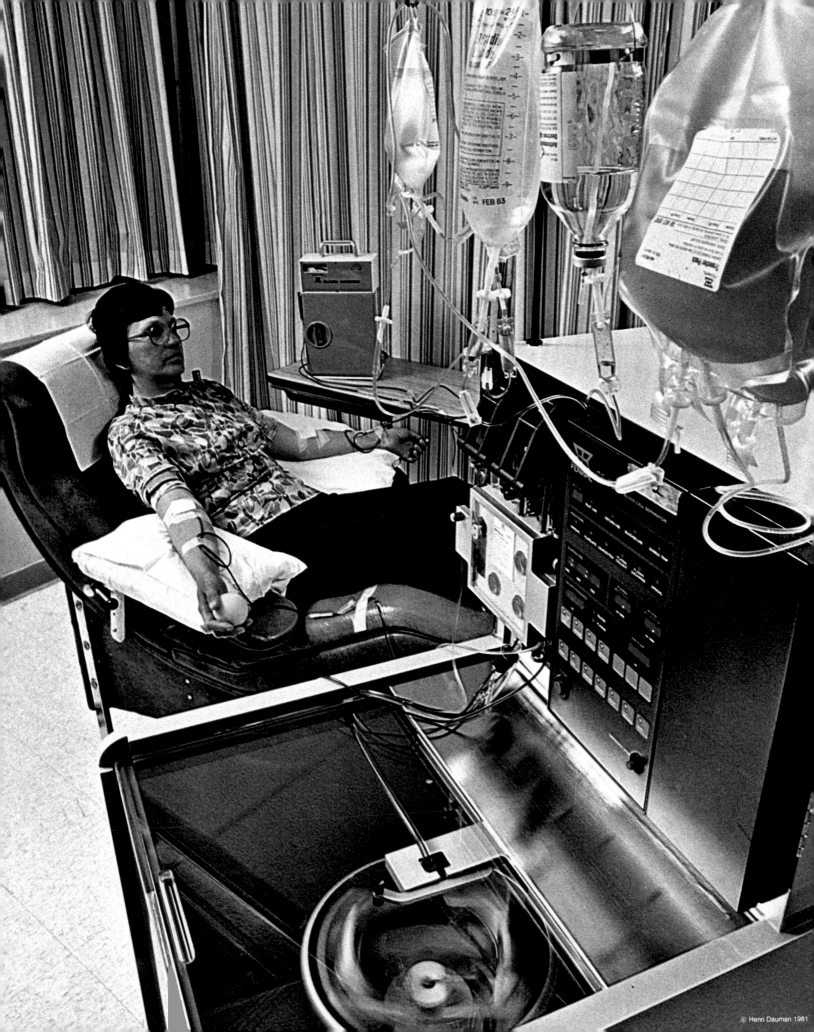

National Institute of Neurological Diseases and Stroke found that an antibody produced by hepatitis patients reacted with an antigen found in the blood of an Australian aborigine. (An antigen is a virus, bacteria or other foreign substance that activates the immune system to produce defensive antibodies.) This antigen proved to be an effective base for a vaccine against infectious hepatitis. Today, vaccines against both types of hepatitis have been formulated.

Antibodies Run Rampant

The immune system normally protects the body against foreign invaders. In lupus, however, it turns against organs and tissues. White blood cells known as lymphocyte B cells begin producing millions of antibodies. Normally, when antibody levels reach a certain point, white cells called suppressor T cells begin to suppress antibody production. In lupus, antibodies multiply unchecked. Soon they adhere to organs, joints and tissues. Some researchers believe lupus causes the immune system to ignore normal safeguards and allows antibodies to target the body's own tissues for destruction.

Some lupus victims experience nothing more than swollen joints. Others suffer fever, fatigue, arthritis, inflammation of the vascular system and kidney disease. Systematic lupus erythematosus (SLE), the most severe form, can attack any part of the body, including the brain and heart. Symptoms can appear intermittently, sometimes at intervals of months or years. It afflicts roughly one in every 500 women and one in every 5,000 men in the United States.

There is no way to determine how severe a lupus patient's symptoms will be. Physicians often prescribe analgesics to help relieve pain. Some patients are also given immune system suppressants to decrease white blood cell activity, although this leaves them vulnerable to viruses and bacterial infections.

A new blood-cleansing technique — apheresis — has been used experimentally to treat severe lupus cases. The patient's blood is siphoned into a large machine where it is spun to separate its components. A membrane filter can then remove targeted portions of the blood according to

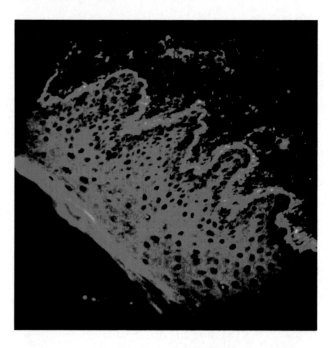

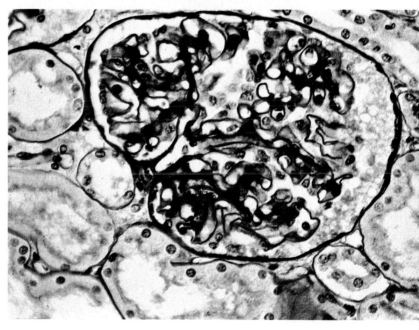

Immune complexes clog renal vessels and disrupt filtering as lupus attacks the kidneys, shown in the biopsy, above. Lupus somehow bypasses immune system safeguards and permits antibodies to turn against tissues.

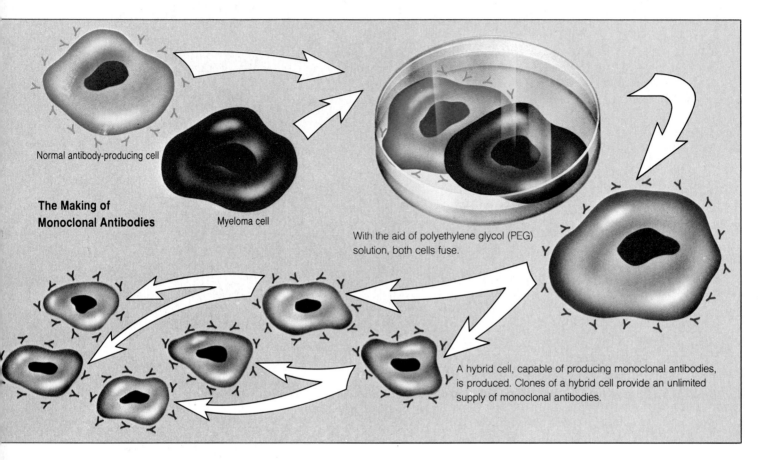

The Making of Monoclonal Antibodies

Normal antibody-producing cell

Myeloma cell

With the aid of polyethylene glycol (PEG) solution, both cells fuse.

A hybrid cell, capable of producing monoclonal antibodies, is produced. Clones of a hybrid cell provide an unlimited supply of monoclonal antibodies.

Monoclonal antibodies, first developed by British scientists George Kohler and Cesar Milstein, may become an important weapon in the fight against cancer and other diseases. The diagram, above, shows how scientists produce these "guided missiles" from a plasma cell and a cancer cell.

their molecular weight. Antibodies or medications can be put into the blood while it is outside the body. One comatose lupus patient regained consciousness after three treatments. Doctors cannot explain why apheresis sometimes brings about remarkable results because they are not certain which of the removed blood components is responsible. Apheresis has also been used to treat other diseases, but with mixed results. All told, between 40,000 and 120,000 patients underwent apheresis in 1980.

Some doctors worry that apheresis might remove cells with long-term immunological memories, which one expert says "might make the patient susceptible to some childhood disease he'd been immune to." Most doctors agree it should be used only on closely monitored hospital patients with chronic progressive diseases.

In 1975, British scientists George Kohler and Cesar Milstein of Cambridge's Medical Research

Council Laboratory of Molecular Biology found what may become an important weapon in the fight against cancer and other diseases. They fused an antibody-producing cell from the spleen of a mouse with a cell from a myeloma, a bone marrow cancer. The product, known as a hybridoma or monoclonal antibody, inherited both the ability to produce antibodies and the ability to thrive. Monoclonal antibodies can clone, or reproduce identical replicas of themselves, endlessly. Because they are antibodies, they can be used as "guided missiles," seeking out and destroying antigens such as viruses, bacteria or cancer cells. Although antigens for cancers have not been identified, monoclonal antibodies derived from cancer cells have been at least partially effective in treating leukemia and cancers of the lymphoid tissues. Scientists hope to devise a way of combining monoclonal antibodies targeted to cancer cells with drugs used in chemotherapy. These substances would destroy cancer cells while leaving normal cells unharmed.

Scientists in various parts of the world are investigating the possibility of using monoclonal antibodies to combat heart disease, immune system disorders and infectious diseases. They are even developing techniques for fighting allergies with monoclonal antibodies. The hybrid cell would theoretically block the action of a targeted allergen. At Harvard Medical School, scientists have used monoclonal antibodies to detect changes in the body chemistry of patients experiencing acute attacks of multiple sclerosis (MS), a disabling disease of the nervous system. Their research suggests MS might be a disorder of the immune system. Other investigators have developed monoclonal antibodies that detect mysterious substances in the blood of leukemic children.

Researchers at Stanford University have fused human bone marrow cancer cells with specially prepared cells from a human spleen to create a pure hybrid cell capable of producing human antibodies. If they succeed in developing this method further, scientists could, at least theoretically, harvest pure antibodies capable of destroying almost any foreign invader for which an antigen can be isolated. Such a breakthrough promises to wipe out countless diseases.

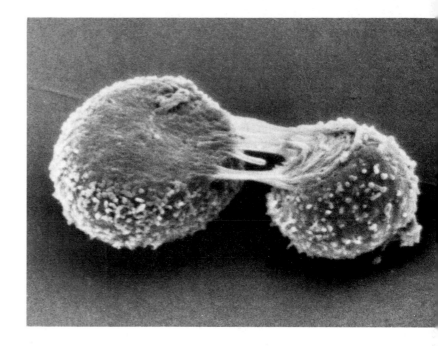

A hybrid cell clones itself, above, creating identical cells capable of reproducing endlessly. The development of monoclonal antibodies from human cells could permit the manufacture of vaccines effective against disease in humans.

Appendix
Vaccinations and Blood Transfusions

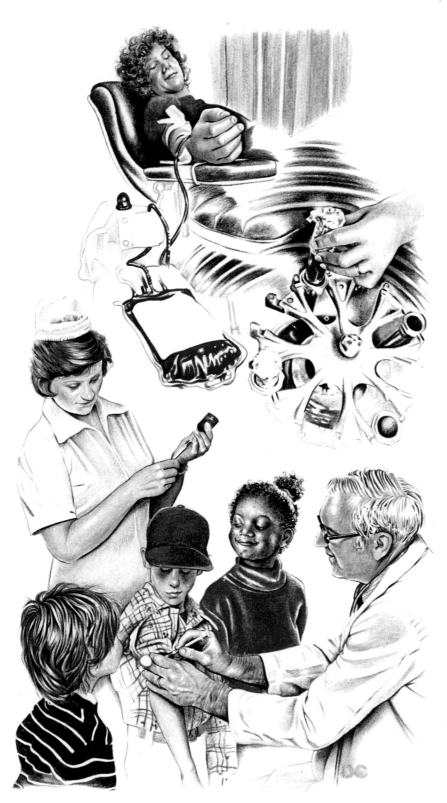

Vaccinations

Smallpox vaccinations are no longer necessary since the disease has been virtually wiped out throughout the world. But polio and other serious diseases are still threats from which only properly immunized children are protected. Health officials hope to eradicate highly contagious childhood illnesses through mass immunization. State requirements can be found on vaccination schedules available at local health departments.

Vaccinations stimulate the body's immune system to produce a mild, controllable form of the disease that stimulates the production of antibodies. These defensive proteins give protection against the full-scale disease.

Side effects from vaccinations are normally very mild, usually little more than a sore arm, slight fever or mild rash. In rare instances, a person may suffer a severe reaction or contract the full-scale disease itself. Persons suffering from diseases affecting the immune system or receiving medications that suppress immunological responses should not receive vaccines made from live viruses like rubella, measles and mumps. Because live virus vaccines can endanger an unborn child, pregnant women and those planning to become pregnant within three months should not receive them. If in doubt, consult a doctor.

Normally, a child needs only one shot for complete protection against measles, mumps and rubella. Diphtheria booster shots should be given every ten years. Tetanus boosters should be administered ten years after an injury that required a remedial dose.

The Centers for Disease Control, part of the U.S. Public Health Service, advises that children receive inoculations at the ages indicated below.

2 months: diphtheria-tetanus-pertussis (D.T.P.)/first dose; oral polio/first dose

4 months: D.T.P./second dose; oral polio/second dose

6 months: D.T.P./third dose

15 months: measles, rubella, mumps

18 months: D.T.P./fourth dose; oral polio/third dose

4 to 6 years: D.T.P./fifth dose; oral polio/fourth dose

14 to 16 years: tetanus-diphtheria booster.

Donating Blood

Each year hospitals in the United States need ten million pints of blood for patients requiring transfusions. Yet only 5 percent of those eligible to give blood actually donate.

Roughly 5 percent of all hospital patients receive transfusions, either for treatment of an illness or to replace blood lost during surgery or through injury or shock.

Requirements for blood donors vary from one blood bank to the next. In general, anyone between age seventeen and sixty-five with a medical history of good health can give. Those over sixty-five who wish to donate need special permission. In some states, seventeen-year-olds need parental consent. Anyone who has suffered from cancer, hepatitis or jaundice cannot donate. Their blood could contain elements harmful to potential blood recipients.

After the initial screening, every donor is given a brief physical examination to determine if weight, body temperature, blood pressure, heart rate and hemoglobin concentration are within acceptable limits.

The donor then reclines on a table or chair where a nurse or technician draws one pint of blood from a vein in his arm. This process takes about ten minutes. After a brief rest, refreshments are served to replace water the body has lost during donation. After eight weeks, the donor may again give blood.

Separating Components

In the laboratory, technicians examine a pilot tube of the donor's blood to confirm blood type and screen for potentially harmful elements.

If the blood meets their requirements, technicians attach three more sterile bags to the pint bag of whole blood. These "satellite bags" will later hold various blood components.

The "quad pack" is run through a centrifuge which spins the blood, separating red blood cells from plasma. A device called a "plasma expressor" then transfers plasma to the second bag. Sealed and cut from the quad pack, the red blood cells are refrigerated and sent to hospitals for use in treating patients with anemia.

The three remaining bags are again placed into the centrifuge, which spins them at a faster rate, forcing platelets to the bottom. The platelet concentrate is essential for blood clotting. It can be used for treating leukemia, cancer and other diseases in which there is a platelet deficiency.

The plasma may be frozen whole and used later for treating a variety of conditions, including coagulation disorders, cirrhosis of the liver and severe burns. In some laboratories, plasma is broken down further through a process known as cryoprecipitation. Technicians place the two remaining bags in a freezer at 80°C. Afterward, the bags are thawed and put in a refrigerator where a clotting factor, known as factor VIII, forms white deposits.

The bags are again centrifuged, forcing the deposits, called cryoprecipitate, to the bottom. This substance is used for treating hemophiliacs who bleed excessively or spontaneously because they lack the clotting factor.

The remaining bag holds a plasma derivative containing proteins such as serum albumin, used in the treatment of shock; globulins, rich in antibodies; and clotting factor concentrates essential to control bleeding caused by plasma protein deficiencies.

Glossary

ABO system the international classification of human blood based on the presence or absence of antigens on red cell membranes.

acid-base balance a state in which the body's production of acid and base equals their outflow.

actin a protein that, along with another protein, is responsible for the contraction and relaxation of muscle.

active immunity the inherent immunologic potential that develops into an ability to produce an immune response to foreign substances.

active transport an energy-requiring process that moves molecules across cell membranes.

adenosine triphosphate ATP; the substance that provides energy for cellular functions.

adrenal glands endocrine glands above each kidney that release the hormones epinephrine and norepinephrine.

agglutination the clumping of antibody-antigen complexes.

agglutinin an antibody circulating in plasma that promotes the clumping of red blood cells.

agglutinogen a substance that stimulates the production of agglutinins.

albumin a protein that circulates in the plasma and acts as a carrier for small molecules.

allele a potentially mutational form of a gene.

allergens an antigen causing an allergic response.

alveoli clustered sacs in the lungs where oxygen and carbon dioxide are exchanged.

amino acids molecules that are the chief components of proteins.

amoeboid moving by the use of pseudopods.

antibiotic an organic compound that inhibits potentially damaging effects of bacteria or toxic substances.

antibody an immunoglobulin protein capable of binding with an antigen.

anticoagulant a substance that delays, inhibits or prevents clotting.

antidiuretic hormone a substance secreted by the posterior portion of the pituitary gland which stimulates reabsorption of water into the circulatory system; vasopressin

antigen a substance that is capable of eliciting an immune response when introduced into the body.

antigen-antibody complex the molecular grouping formed when an antibody binds to an antigen.

antigenic determinants the sites on an antigen which activate lymphocytes; a group of amino acids or sugar residues that identify an antigen as foreign material.

antitoxin a substance that neutralizes poisonous material.

apheresis a method of cleansing the blood and filtering out certain components.

arteriole a small artery.

artery a vessel conveying blood away from the heart.

atom the smallest particle of a chemical element.

attenuate to render a virus less potent.

autoimmune disease a disorder of the immune system in which antibodies are directed against the body's own tissues.

bacterium a one-cell organism lacking membrane-bound internal structures.

baroreceptors nerve endings in the walls of blood vessels that monitor changes in blood pressure.

basophil a type of white blood cell possessing granules that tint blue when stained with biological dyes.

B cell a lymphocyte that produces antibodies and confers humoral immunity.

bicarbonate buffer a mixture of carbonic acid and sodium bicarbonate that regulates the acid-base balance in the body.

bile a yellowish liquid secreted by the liver which aids in digestion.

bilirubin a bile pigment derived from the destruction of hemoglobin.

bloodletting the practice of removing blood from veins for therapeutic reasons.

blood pressure a measurable force generated by heart contractions that maintains blood flow in the circulatory system.

bone marrow a soft substance which fills the bone cavity; site of blood cell production.

botulinum bacterium an agent causing food poisoning in man.

bronchi the paired tubes that branch into the lungs.

bursa of Fabricius a saclike organ in the intestinal region of chickens to which lymphocytes migrate for maturation into B cells.

Cambrian era a period of geologic history ranging from 570 to 500 million years ago.

cancer a malignant tumor or abnormal growth that can spread throughout the body.

capillaries minute blood vessels that connect arterioles and venules.

carbohydrates compounds, such as sugar, which constitute a major source of animal food.

carotid artery a large blood vessel in the neck which supplies blood to the brain via the systemic system.

cartilage fibrous material attached to the surfaces of bones.

cell the structural and functional unit of an organism composed of cytoplasm and usually containing a nucleus and, in animals, surrounded by a membrane.

cell-mediated immunity specific immunity resulting from T lymphocyte activity.

cell membrane the outermost covering of a cell; plasma membrane.

chain a linear arrangement of atoms.

chemoreceptors sense organs that are sensitive to changes in the chemical composition of blood.

chemotactic factor a lymphokine which chemically attracts phagocytes and leukocytes to the site of infection.

chemotaxis the biochemical message that increases the migration of cells toward a specific site.

chemotherapy treating diseases with chemical agents; drug therapy.

cholera a fatal infectious viral disease characterized by severe diarrhea, muscle cramps and vomiting.

chromosome threads of genetic material that contain the hereditary code.

circulatory system the pathways through which blood and lymph travel throughout the body.

clone a cell derived from one identical parent cell.

clotting factors essential substances circulating in the blood which mediate the process of clotting.

clotting time the time required for blood to coagulate in a glass tube.

coagulation the formation of a clot.

collagen a fibrous protein found in

bone, cartilage and connective tissue.

complement system   a series of at least nine serum proteins that aid T and B cells in the immune response.

connective tissue   a collection of functionally similar cells that protect and support nerves, glands and muscles.

corpuscle   a red or white blood cell.

cytoplasm   the protoplasm exclusive of the nucleus in which most chemical activity occurs.

delayed hypersensitivity   a cell-mediated immune response that results hours after exposure to antigen.

dendritic macrophage   the specific name given to a macrophage in the lymph nodes.

deoxyribonucleic acid   DNA; the double helix of genetic material in which hereditary characteristics bond.

dialysis   the separation of smaller molecules from larger ones in an attempt to cleanse a solution of undesired material.

diffusion   the passage of molecules from a region of high concentration to a region of low concentration.

diphtheria   an infectious disease characterized by the formation of a membrane over the air passage.

diploid   containing two sets of chromosomes.

edema   swelling due to accumulation of fluid.

electron   a subatomic particle.

embolism   the blockage of a vessel by a dislodged clot.

endocrine gland   a ductless gland that secretes hormones into the circulatory system.

endocrine system   the organs and other structures that release hormones into the circulatory system to influence metabolism and other bodily processes.

endocytosis   the absorption of molecules too large to pass freely across the cell membrane.

endothelial cells   cells lining the interior surface of blood vessels and lymphatics.

enzyme   a protein molecule that enhances or accelerates a chemical reaction.

eosinophil   a type of white blood cell possessing granules that tint red when stained with biological dyes.

epinephrine   a hormone produced by the adrenal gland's medulla which functions to increase blood pressure

and heart rate; adrenalin.

erythrocyte   a red blood cell.

erythropoetin   a hormone produced by the kidneys and liver that signals the production of red blood cells.

extracellular fluid   the body fluids found outside the cells.

extrinsic pathway   the clot-forming mechanism initiated when blood contacts damaged vessels or tissues surrounding blood vessels.

fibrin   the protein that forms the essential portion of a blood clot.

fibrinogen   the inactive form of a coagulation protein converted to fibrin during clot formation.

fibrinolysis   the breakdown of a clot by enzymes.

fibrin stabilizing factor   a blood component that strengthens fibrin threads.

fibrous protein   an insoluble structural protein.

forbidden clone   an undesired clone which can cause a deleterious auto-immune response.

gamma globulin   one of four major groups of serum proteins which contain the antibodies.

gene   a unit of hereditary information located on the chromosomes.

genetic marker   a gene or substance that can be used diagnostically as an indicator of hereditary disorder.

gestation   the period of a fetus's development in the uterus.

gland   a specialized organ that releases secretions.

globulin   a group of proteins circulating in the plasma.

glomerulus   a tuft of capillaries within the kidney.

glucose   the most abundant type of sugar found in animals; a monosaccharide.

granules   insoluble particles found in cytoplasm.

granulocyte   any cell displaying granules in its cytoplasm.

haploid   containing only one set of chromosomes.

hapten   a foreign particle or substance too small to initiate an immune response of its own.

heavy chain   the larger of the two types of strings of atoms that make up an immunoglobulin molecule.

helper T cells   a subgroup of T lym-

phocytes which aid B cells to mature into antibody-producing plasma cells.

hematologist   one who specializes in the study of blood.

hematology   the study of blood and blood-forming tissues.

heme   the iron-containing component of hemoglobin responsible for oxygen transport.

hemoglobin   the iron-containing molecule of red blood cells responsible for oxygen and carbon dioxide transport.

hemolytic anemia   a disorder characterized by an increased rate of red blood cell destruction.

hemophilia   a genetic disease characterized by the failure of blood to clot.

hemorrhage   loss of blood; bleeding.

heparin   a potent anticoagulant in lung and liver tissue.

hepatic vein   the vein in the liver that conveys blood toward the heart.

hereditary   transmitted from parent to offspring; genetic.

heterozygote   an organism that carries two different alleles on at least one gene.

high-zone tolerance   a condition in which antigen levels are so high that the immune system cannot respond adequately.

histamine   a crystalline compound that stimulates gastric secretions and dilates blood vessels.

histocompatibility antigen   a genetically determined substance normally found on cell membranes that stimulates production of an antibody; used medically to determine the compatibility of tissues in transplants.

homeostasis   the maintenance of the body's internal environment in a balanced state.

homozygote   an organism that carries identical alleles on one gene.

hormones   chemical messengers of the body produced by glands of the endocrine system.

humoral immunity   resistance to a specific disease provided by B cells and their antibodies.

humors   the fluids or semifluids in the body which were historically believed to affect mental disposition and health.

hybrid   the offspring from two parents that differ in one or more genetic characteristics.

hypothalamus the portion of the brain that maintains a homeostatic environment throughout the organism.

idiotype antigenic determinants which compose distinguishing characteristics among antibodies.

immediate hypersensitivity an antibody-mediated response characterized by increased vascular permeability and smooth muscle contraction.

immune having a special resistance to specific disease.

immune system a composite of proteins and cells that help fight infective agents and disease.

immunize to protect from disease by vaccination or inoculation.

immunoglobulins antibodies responsible for conferring immunity.

inflammation a localized immune reaction characterized by swelling, redness and pain.

influenza the flu; a highly contagious viral disease causing inflamed nasal and bronchial passages.

interstitial fluid the liquid in which cells are bathed.

interstitium the spaces between the cells of body tissues.

intracellular fluid liquid and dissolved substances found within the cell.

intraoperative autotransfusion the injection of a patient's own blood during surgery.

intrinsic factor a natural substance which confers the ability to absorb vitamin B_{12}.

intrinsic pathway the clot-forming mechanism initiated by damage to the blood itself.

ion an electrically charged atom or molecule formed by the loss or gain of at least one electron.

jaundice a condition in which excess bile pigment accumulates in the tissues, tinting the skin yellow.

kidney an organ which regulates the amount of water in the system, the substances in the blood and the amount of urine excreted.

killer T cell a cell that causes the destruction of specific antigenic cells.

Kupffer's cell a macrophage cell located in the liver.

larva an immature form of an animal which differs significantly from the adult form.

leukemia malignant diseases affecting the blood-forming organs characterized by abnormally high levels of white blood cells.

leukocytes white blood cells produced in the bone marrow.

light chain the shorter of the two types of strings of atoms that make up an immunoglobulin molecule.

lipid a fatty substance that is insoluble in water and body fluids.

low-zone tolerance a condition in which the amount of antigen introduced to the immune system is insufficient to elicit an immune response.

lymph the blood cells and liquid absorbed from the spaces between cells and returned to the circulatory system, after being filtered by the lymph nodes.

lymphatic system the system that transports nutrients and lymph back to the blood stream.

lymph nodes masses of spongy tissue that supply lymphocytes to the circulatory system and remove foreign particles from lymph.

lymphocyte mononuclear white blood cell comprising B cells and T cells.

lymphokines effector substances released by T lymphocytes which aid in immune response.

lysis the death of a cell caused by the destruction of the cell membrane.

lysosomes vacuoles within a cell that contain degradation enzymes.

macrophage "big eater"; the most potent type of phagocytic cell in the blood stream.

macrophage activation factor a lymphokine capable of inducing macrophages to enlarge and consume at an excelled rate in the face of an immune response.

malignant having a progressively worsening course.

medulla the inner core of an organ or structure.

medulla oblongata the area in the back of the brain which controls respiration.

megakaryocyte a large cell of the bone marrow from which platelets arise.

memory cells cells produced from an activated clone of lymphocytes endowed with the memory to fight a specific antigen upon its reintroduction to the immune system.

menarche the onset of menstruation.

menstruation periodic discharge of blood due to hormone-regulated changes that shed the lining of the uterus.

metabolism a chemical reaction occurring within a cell or organism.

metarteriole a small artery that links arterioles to capillaries.

microbes microscopic organisms.

migration inhibition factor a lymphokine which, when released by T cells, slows further migration of leukocytes from the scene of an infection.

molecule the smallest unit of any compound consisting of at least two atoms.

monoclonal antibody an antibody produced by the fusion of a normal B cell and a cell from a myeloma.

monocytes mononuclear phagocytes formed in the bone marrow and transported to tissues where they develop into macrophages.

monomer a single molecule capable of linking with other molecules to form a polymer.

mononuclear cell a cell with a kidney-shaped nucleus that fills most of the cell's interior.

mutation an inheritable change in genetic information.

myeloma uncontrolled production of bone marrow cells; a bone marrow tumor.

myosin a principal protein component of muscles that make up thick filaments.

nephron the basic functional unit of the kidney.

neutrophil the most abundant type of white blood cell.

norepinephrine a powerful hormone that contracts arteries and capillaries; noradrenalin.

nucleus the part of a cell which contains the genetic information in the form of DNA.

organ a part of the body consisting of tissues grouped to form a structural and functional unit.

organic pertaining to living things; compounds containing carbon.

osmosis the movement of water from an area of high concentration to an area of low concentration.

osmotic pressure a measurement of the differences of two solutions separated by a penetrable membrane.

oxidation the gaining of oxygen by the

loss of hydrogen; the formation of an ion by the loss of an electron.

oxyhemoglobin   the molecule formed by the binding of oxygen to hemoglobin.

partial pressure   the pressure exerted by an individual gas in a mixture of gases.

passive immunity   the transference of foreign leukocytes to the blood stream for the purpose of passing the immunity of one individual to another.

pH   the value representing acidity or alkalinity of a solution.

phagocytes   cells that ingest dead cells, foreign particles and debris floating throughout the body.

phagocytosis   the act of engulfing cells and debris by phagocytes.

phagosome   an intercellular capsule encompassing debris ingested through phagocytosis.

pituitary gland   a two-lobed organ in the brain which secretes hormones.

plague   a highly contagious and deadly bacterial disease.

plasma   the fluid portion of blood containing proteins, minerals and salts.

plasma cell   a mature B lymphocyte capable of producing antibodies.

platelets   structures found in blood that play a major role in clotting.

polymer   a large molecule made by the fusion of small molecules known as monomers.

polymerization   the formation of a complex compound from simple molecules.

polymorphonuclear cell   a cell with a nucleus that assumes many shapes.

polypeptide   a large molecule consisting of at least two amino acids bonded together.

portal vein   a large vessel carrying blood from the intestines to the liver.

precapillary sphincter   a ringlike muscle that can control the flow of blood to capillaries.

pressure   the force exerted on a surface relative to a given area.

prostaglandins   a group of naturally produced fatty acids that stimulate the contraction of smooth muscles.

protein   organic compounds containing nitrogen; a major constituent of living cells.

protoplasm   the jellylike substance in which most cellular activity occurs.

pseudopods   temporary cytoplasmic extensions produced by cells for purposes of locomotion and for engulfing material.

pulmonary circulation   the circular course of blood to the lungs where the exchange of carbon dioxide for oxygen occurs.

putrefaction   the decomposition of proteins resulting from microorganism activity.

radiation therapy   the exposure of tissue to X-rays for the purpose of destroying cancerous cells.

radioimmunoassay   a test for measuring the presence of a substance in the blood.

respiration   the process of inhaling oxygen and exhaling carbon dioxide.

Rh factor   the most complex group of blood types.

rubriblast   the first recognizable precursor of mature red blood cells.

secretion   the release of a substance by cells.

serotonin   a substance produced in the body that constricts blood vessels.

serum   the clear component of animal blood which separates into liquid and solid elements.

shock   a condition characterized by inadequate blood supply to the body tissues due to massive loss of blood or the inability of the heart to pump blood efficiently.

sickling crisis   an acute attack of sickle cell anemia which can debilitate children, causing stroke and seizure, and can also leave adult organs susceptible to dysfunction.

sinusoid   large, merging vessels found in the liver.

smallpox   a viral disease causing fever and bodily lesions.

smooth muscle   nonstriated musculature.

stem cell   a cell produced in the bone marrow which proliferates and divides to produce a progeny of leukocytes.

suppressor T cells   a subgroup of T lymphocytes helping to inhibit antibody production of B cells.

surface area   the outer or topmost area of tissue.

systemic system   the portion of the circulatory system excluding the lungs.

T cell   a lymphocyte that can kill tumor and transplant-tissue cells.

tetanus   a fatal infectious bacterial disease causing muscle spasms.

thrombosis   the formation of a clot that might obstruct normal blood flow.

thymic hormone   a substance released by the thymus that enhances the maturation of lymphocytes.

thymus gland   an organ located behind the breastbone important in the development of cell-mediated immune responses.

tissue histiocyte   a macrophage found in tissue beneath the skin.

toxin   a poisonous substance.

transfer factor   a substance capable of activating other T cells necessary to aid in an immune response.

transfusion   the injection of whole blood or its components into the blood stream.

tuberculosis   a deadly infectious bacterial disease affecting the lungs in man.

tumor   a progressive and uncontrollable growth of tissue.

universal donor   a person with type O blood, a blood group which can be transfused to any individual without complication.

universal recipient   a person able to receive any type of blood without complication.

urushiol   the allergen in poison ivy.

uterus   muscular organ in which the fetus develops.

vaccine   a preparation of weakened or killed viral or bacterial material which, once injected, confers immunity to that particular virus.

vascularization   the process or development of vessels in the system.

vasoconstrictor   a substance that causes the blood vessels to constrict.

vein   a vessel that carries blood toward the heart.

venule   a small vein.

vertigo   a sensation of dizziness due to an inner ear or central nervous system disorder.

villi   fingerlike projections found on the interior surface of the small intestine where water and nutrients are absorbed.

virus   an infective noncellular particle composed of genetic material.

vivisection   the dissection of a living animal.

zymogen   an inactive precursor of an enzyme.

Photographic Credits

Introduction
6, Manfred Kage/Peter Arnold, Inc.

A Living Symbol
8, Adolph Gottlieb, *Thrust*. The Metropolitan Museum of Art, George A. Hearn Fund, 1959. 10, Annan Photo Features. 11, Nicolas Poussin, *Baccanale*. SCALA/Editorial Photocolor Archives. 12, (left) The Granger Collection, New York. 12-13, Justus of Ghent, *The Communion of the Apostles*, SCALA/Editorial Photocolor Archives. 13, (right) Sipa/ Black Star. 14, Mary Evans Picture Library. 15, The Bettmann Archive. 16, Mary Evans Picture Library. 17, George Morland, *The End of the Hunt*. National Gallery of Art, Washington, D.C., Widener Collection. 18, Goya, *The Family of Charles IV*. Copyright © Museo del Prado, Madrid. All rights reserved. Partial or total reproduction is prohibited. 19, Sonia Halliday Photographs. 21, (left) The British Library (right) Courtesy of the Freer Gallery of Art, Smithsonian Institution, Washington, D.C. 22, The Granger Collection, New York. 23, (top) The British Library (bottom) Adriaen Brouwer, *The Village Barber-Surgeon*. The Granger Collection, New York. 24, 25, The Bettmann Archive. 26, **Thomas B. Allen.** 27, Jacques Louis David, *Antoine-Laurent Lavoisier and His Wife*. The Metropolitan Museum of Art, Purchase, Mr. and Mrs. Charles Wrightsman Gift, 1977.

The Liquid Tissue
28, Morgan Russell, *Cosmic Synchromy*, Munson-Williams-Proctor Institute, Utica, NY. 30, **Mark Seidler.** 32, Manfred Kage/Peter Arnold, Inc. 33, Alfred Owczarzak/Taurus Photos. Foldout, (outside) © Alfred T. Lamme, 1976 (inside) **Ken Goldammer.** 34, (top) Animals, Animals/Oxford Scientific Films (bottom) © Animals, Animals/ Stouffer Enterprises, Inc. 35, (top) S. C. Bisserot /Bruce Coleman, Inc. (bottom) Jeff Rotman/Peter Arnold, Inc. 36, Manfred Kage/Peter Arnold, Inc. 37, (left) Lennart Nilsson from his book *Behold Man*, published in the U.S. by Little, Brown & Co., Boston (right) from *Corpuscles* by Marcel Bessis. Springer-Verlag, Berlin, New York © 1974. 38, **Mark Seidler** from *Biology* by C. K. Levy. Goodyear Publishing Co. 39, © Gabe Palmer/The Image Bank. 40, from *Corpuscles* by Marcel Bessis. Springer-Verlag, Berlin, New York © 1974. 41, © John Watney Photo Library. 42, BBC Hulton Picture Library. 43, (left) Sonia Halliday Photographs (right) Courtesy of the Freer Gallery of Art, Smithsonian Institution, Washington, D.C. 44, The Bettmann Archive. 45, Ann Ronan Picture Library. 46, (top & middle) Runk/ Schoenberger from Grant Heilman (bottom) **Jack Lanza.** 47, **Thomas B. Allen.** 49, **Nancy Van Meter.** 50, **Thomas B. Allen.** 51, (top) **Jennifer**

Arnold (right middle) © Dennis Stock-/Magnum (right bottom) © M. Isy-Schwart/The Image Bank. 52, The Bettmann Archive. 53, Edith O. Haun-/Stock Boston.

The Great Exchange
54, from *Aladdin*, illustrated by Errol Le Cain (Viking Press, New York). Illustration reprinted by permission of Faber and Faber, Ltd. 57, **Lewis E. Calver.** 58, Biophoto Associates. 59, **Joyce Hurwitz.** 60, **Mark Seidler.** 61, (both) Biophoto Associates. 63, **George V. Kelvin.** 64, **Lewis E. Calver.** 65, Lennart Nilsson from his book *Behold Man*, published in the U.S. by Little, Brown & Co., Boston. 66, **Thomas B. Allen.** 67, (left) Gamma/ Liaison (right) © Armando Jenik/The Image Bank. 68, Biophoto Associates. 69, National Library of Medicine. 70, **Lewis E. Calver.** 71, Biophoto Associates/Paul Wheater. 73, Manfred Kage/ Peter Arnold, Inc.

Self-Healing Fabric
74, Österreichisches Museum für Angewandte Kunst, Vienna, by permission of Verlag Galerie Welz Salzberg. 76, Dr. James White, University of Minnesota. 77, (left) Courtesy of Dr. Jerome Gross, Massachusetts General Hospital (right) Manfred Kage/Peter Arnold, Inc. 78, **Virginia L. Schoonover.** 79, E. Bernstein and E. Kairinen, Gillette Research Institute. 80, **Thomas B. Allen.** 81, FPG/Arthur M. Siegelman. 83, **Jane Gordon.** 85, (both) FPG/Arthur M. Siegelman. 86, Bernard P. Wolff/Photo Researchers, Inc. 87, SCALA/Editorial Photocolor Archives. 88, (both) Courtesy of Abbott Laboratories. 89, The Granger Collection, New York. 90, The Lord Chamberlain's Office, London, England. 91, **Karen Karlsson.** 92, BBC Hulton Picture Library. 93, Culver Pictures. 94, Mary Evans Picture Library. 95, Yale-New Haven Hospital.

A Mobilized Army
96, Henri Matisse, *Ivy in Flower*. Dallas Museum of Fine Arts, Foundation for the Arts Collection, Gift of the Albert and Mary Lasker Foundation. 98, The Bettmann Archive. 99, (top) National Library of Medicine (bottom) The Bettmann Archive. 100, (top) BBC Hulton Picture Library (bottom) John Moss/ Black Star. 101, **Thomas B. Allen.** 102, (left) Jan Henson, National Jewish Hospital/National Asthma Center (right) from *Tissues and Organs* by Richard G. Kessel and Randy H. Kardon. W. H. Freeman and Company © 1979. 103, National Library of Medicine. 104, Dr. Victor A. Najjar, Tufts University Medical School, Boston, MA. 105, (left) from Malech, Root, and Gallin, "Structural Analysis of Human Neutrophil Migration," *Journal of Cell Biology*, 75:666–693 (1977) (right) **John R. Murphy.** 106,

Thomas B. Allen. 107, (top) Mayer Goren, Ph.D., National Jewish Hospital/ National Asthma Center (bottom) **Virginia L. Schoonover.** 108, **John R. Murphy.** 109, Biophoto Associates. 110, National Library of Medicine. 111, **Lou Bory & Associates** (inset) from *Tissues and Organs* by Richard G. Kessel and Randy H. Kardon. W. H. Freeman and Company © 1979. 112, (top) Dr. David R. Davies and Dr. Louis W. Labaw, National Institutes of Health (bottom) **Esperance Shatarah.** 113, **Sam Haltom/ Another Color.** 114-115, **Karen Karlsson.** 115, (right) Lennart Nilsson from his book *Behold Man*, published in the U.S. by Little, Brown & Co., Boston. 116, **Virginia L. Schoonover.** 117, **Virginia L. Schoonover.** 118, James de Leon, Jr., photographer, Texas Children's Hospital, Houston. 119, Victor Lorian, M.D., Chairman, Microbiology and Epidemiology, Bronx-Lebanon Hospital and Professor of Laboratory Medicine, Albert Einstein College of Medicine. 120, (top) FPG/Heiselmann (bottom) Copyright © 1981 by David Scharf. All rights reserved. 121, Copyright © 1978 by David Scharf. All rights reserved. 122, National Jewish Hospital/National Asthma Center. 123, John P. Caulfield and Ann Hein, Harvard Medical School, from *The Journal of Cell Biology*. 124, **Nancy Van Meter.** 127, (both) Andrejs Liepins, Ph.D., Memorial University of Newfoundland, Canada.

Perils of the River
128, Biophoto Associates/Paul Wheater. 130, from *Flora auf Deutschland* by Otto W. Thome, 1889. Courtesy of The Library of Congress. 131, Martha Holmes/ TIME Magazine. 132, from *Corpuscles* by Marcel Bessis. Springer-Verlag, Berlin, New York © 1974. 133, **Adolphe Brotman.** 134, (both) Prof. M. I. Barnhart, Wayne State University School of Medicine, Detroit, MI. 135, **Nancy Van Meter.** 136,137, **Jennifer Arnold.** 138, FPG/Arthur M. Siegelman. 139, **Sam Haltom/Another Color.** 140, St. Jude Children's Research Hospital, Memphis, TN. 141, (both) Photri. 142, (top) Courtesy of Bruce Wetzel, Esther Kendig, Harry Schaefer, National Cancer Institute, Bethesda, MD (bottom) Johns Hopkins Medical Institutions. 143, Fritz Goro. 144, 145, © 1980 Huntington Potter & David Dressler/Life Picture Service. 145, (bottom) Wadley Institutes of Molecular Medicine, Dallas, TX. 146, (both) Fredrik D. Bodin. 147, **Mitchell Kuff.** 148, © Henri Dauman, 1981/*Medical World News.* 149, (both) David Koffler, M.D., 1980. 150, **Karen Karlsson.** 151, Copyright © 1980 by David Scharf. All rights reserved.

Appendix
152, **Donald Gates.**

Index

Page numbers in bold type indicate location of illustrations.

fungus, 40
Funke, Otto, 45

G

Gajdusek, D. Carlton, 147
Galen (Galenus, Claudius), 20, 24, 25
gamma globulin, *see* globulin
gastrointestinal
    cancer, 130
    tract, **57**, 113
gene, 49, 90, 91, 92, 118, 129–30, **133**, 136,
    142
genetic marker, 130
genetic trait, 51
George IV, **91**
German measles, *see* disease, rubella
Gilfillan, Seabury, 132
gladiator, 42
globulin, 30, 70, 79, 153
    alpha, 30
    beta, 30
    gamma, 30, 112
glomerulus, 71, 72
glucose, 62, 69, 70
glucose-6-phosphate dehydrogenase,
    129
glycogen, 70
glycoprotein, 131
granule, **105**, 109
granulocyte, 102
Green, Saul, 144
"green sickness," *see* disease, chlorosis

H

hapten, 123
Harvey, William, 25, 27, 42, 43
hay fever, *see* allergy
health, symbol of, 9, 18
heart, 19, 20, 25, 42, 56, 59, 60, 62, 65, 70,
    81, 108, 111, 149
    attack, 81, 88, 137
    disease, 81, **83**, 130, 151
    failure, *see* heart attack
Heinrich, **91**
Hellem, Arvid, 84,
hematology, 46, 80, 81, 84
heme, 37–38, **38**
hemoglobin, 31, 37, 38, 45, 50, 65, 66, 67,
    69, 76, 129, 132, 136, 153,
hemophilia, *see* disease
hemorrhage, 43, 45, 78, 82, 84, 86, 88, 90,
    91, 92, **133**
hemostatic plug, 79
heparin, *see* drug
hepatic artery, *see* artery, hepatic
hepatitis, *see* disease
    vaccine, 147, 149
heredity, 90, 119
Herophilus, 20
Hewson, William, 80
Hippocrates, 19, 20, 30, 31, 39
histamine, 107, 108, **108**, 120, 123, 125,
    126

histiocyte, 105
Hoagland, Robert, 139
Holy Grail, 14
homeostasis, 56, **57**, 60, 69, 70
Hoppe-Seyler, Felix, 45
hormone, 7, 29, **30**, 31, 39, **60**, 61, 81, 102,
    110, 130
hot blood, 17
Howell, W. H., 81
human leukocyte antigen (H.L.A.), 48
humor, 19–20, 21, 43, 109
humoral immunity, 109
Huygens, Constantijn, 26
hybridoma, *see* monoclonal antibody
hydrogen, 37, 50, 69
    ions, 72
    peroxide, 103
hydroxide ions, 69
hypercoagulability, 81–82
hypersensitivity reaction, 123

I

idiotype, 118
Iliad, 16
Imhotep, 19
immune complex, 149
immune response, **114–15,** 119
immune system, 48, 49, 100, 102, 109,
    112, 113, 118, 119–20, 124, 125, 126,
    127, 142, 144, 149, 151, 152
    suppressant, 149
immunity, 40, 98, 101, 102, 114, 118,
    122–23, 126, 139–40,
    active, 119
    passive, 119
immunoglobulin, *see also* globulin,
    gamma
    IgA, 112
    IgD, 112
    IgE, 112, 119–20, 123
    IgG, 112–13, 114, **114–15, 117,** 119, 123
    IgM, 112–13, 114, 119
immunoglobulin therapy, 144
immunological memory, 150
infection, 97, 98, 99, 101, 105, 107, 113,
    119, 126, 136, 141, 147, 151
infectious mononucleosis, *see* disease
inflammation, 100, 102, 107, 108, 109,
    114, **117, 124**
inoculation, 101
intercellular fluid, 103
interferon, *see* drug
internal infection, 132
interstitial fluid, 55, 60, 61, 67, 108
interstitium, 61
intestine, 56, 66, 69, 70, 82, 105, **133**
    small, 70, 110
intracellular fluid, 61, 71
intraoperative autotransfusion, 52
intrinsic clotting pathway, 78, 79
intrinsic factor, **133**, 135
ions, 69, 71
iron, 7, 37–38, 39, 45, 50, 133, **133**

iron deficiency anemia, *see* disease,
    anemia
iron lung, 106

J

Janssen, Zacharias, 27
jaundice, *see* disease
Jefferson, Thomas, 16
Jenner, Edward, 98, 99, 101
Jesus, 42, 43

K

Kan, Yuet Wai, 135–36
Kasim, Abul, 88
kidney, 56, 59, 71, 72, 87, 135, 140, 147,
    149
Kirby, James, 84
"kissing disease," *see* disease, infectious
    mononucleosis
Koagulation-Vitamin, *see* vitamin, K
Koch, Robert, 99
Kohler, George, 150
kosher meat, 10
Krim, Mathilde, 144, 147
Kupffer's cell, 105

L

lacteal, 110
Landsteiner, Karl, 45, 46, 47
Lavoisier, Antoine Laurent, 27, 45
lead poisoning, 131–32
lecithin, **83**, 84, 87
Leeuwenhoek, Anton van, 25, 26, 27
leprosy, 17
leukemia, *see* disease
leukocyte, *see* blood cell, leukocyte
Liepins, Andrejs, 127
life (force), 9, 11, 14, 15, 18, 19, 41, 55, 62,
    66, 69
ligature, 25
light microscope, 76
lineage, 17
Link, Karl Paul, 86
lipid, 61, 62, **63**
liver, 19, 20, 31, 56, **70**, 72, 73, 82, **83**,
    84–85, 86, 88, 105, 107, 140, 144, 147,
    153
loop of Henle, 71
Lower, Richard, 43–44
Luise, **91**
lung, 27, 29, 37, 38, 39, 55, 56, **57**, 62, 65,
    67, 69, 81, 82, 87, 105, 135
lupus, *see* disease
lymph, 108, 110, 112, **117**, 126
    gland, 40, 41, 80
    node, 31, 105, **108**, 109, 110, 111, **111**,
        113, 116
    vessel, 69, 80, **111**
lymphatic system, 70
lymphocyte, *see also* blood cell, leuko-
    cyte
    B cell, 109, 110, 112, 113, 114, **114–15,**
        116, 118–19, 123, 124, **124,** 125, 126,
        149

T cell, 109, 110, 113, 114, **114–15**, 116, 118–19, 123, 124, **124**, 125, 126, 127
lymphoid tissue, 151
lymphokine, 116, 118, 123, 126
lysosome, 107, 109

M
macrophage, *see* blood cell
macrophage chemotactic factor (MCF), *see* lymphokine
Magendie, François, 66
magnesium, 61
malaria, *see* disease
Malpighi, Marcello, 26, 27, 59
margination, **108**, 109
Masai, 9
mast cell, 82, 107, **108**, 120, 122, 123
measles, *see* disease
Medea, 42
megakaryocyte, 77
membrane, 61, 62, **63**, 72, **117**
    respiratory, 62
Mendel, Gregor, 90
menstruation, 14–15, **133**
mercury, 50
metabolism, 31, 71
metals, 31
metarterioles, 56, 59, **59**
Metchnikoff, Elie, 100, 102
microbe, 99, 101
microorganism, 7, 25, 26, 99, 102, 107, 108, 109, 113, 116
microscope, 20, 25, 26, 27, 39, 46, 81, 102, 109
milieu intérieur, 55, 66
Milstein, Cesar, 150
mineral, 7, 30, 31, 62, 70, 71
miracle, 12, 19
monoblast, 107, **107**
monoclonal antibody, **150**, 151
monocyte, *see* blood cell, leukocyte
monomer, 79
mononucleosis, *see* disease, infectious mononucleosis
Motulsky, Arno G., 129–30
mouth, 62, 71
mucous membrane, 108, 112
multiple myeloma, *see* disease
multiple sclerosis (MS), *see* disease
mumps, *see* disease
mutation, 91, 118, 126, 136, 147
myeloma, *see* disease
myocardial infarction, *see* heart, attack
myosin, 79

N
National Blood Bank, 52
National Blood Transfusion Committee, 52
nephron, 71
nerve fiber, 59
nervous system, 59
neutrophil, *see* blood cell, leukocyte

nitrogen, 37, 38, 50, 62
nonspecific immunity, 108
norepinephrine, 59
nose, 62, 108
nucleus, 31, 37, 71, 77, 105, 109, 125, **139**

O
oral contraceptive, 133
Osler, Sir William, 76
Ottenberg, Reuben, 46
Otto, John C., 88, 90
Owren, Paul, 84
oxidation, 62
oxygen, 29, 31, **32**, 33, 37, 38–39, **38**, 45, 50, 55, 56, 59, 60, **60**, 62, **64**, 65, 66, 67, 69, 108, 129, **133**, 135, 136–37
oxyhemoglobin, 65

P
pancreas, 66
Paracelsus, 15
parasite, 40, 41
Paré, Ambroise, 24, 25
Passover, 10, 12
Pasteur, Louis, 99, 101
Patterson, Clair C., 132
penicillin, *see* drug
peptic ulcer, 88, 130
peptide, 79
peritoneum, 72
permeability, 60, 61, 72, 107
pernicious anemia, *see* disease, anemia
pertussis, *see* disease
Perutz, Max, 50
pH, 69, 72
phagocyte, *see* blood cell, leukocyte
phagocytosis, 40, 102, 105, **105**, 115, 126
phagosome, 103, 104, 105, **105**
phlebitis, 82
phlebotomy, *see* bloodletting
phosphate, 61
placenta, **49**, 95
plasma, 30, **30**, 37, 46, 52, 55, 71, 72, 77, 79, 80, 90–95, 113, **114–15**, 125, 126, 139, 153
    protein, 30–31, 61, 70, 72, 94, 153
plasmin, 82, **83**, 85, 88
plasminogen, 82, **83**, 88
plasminogen activator, 82, **83**, 87
platelet, *see* blood cell
    adhesiveness index (PAI), **83**, 84
Plato, 80
Pliny, 22
pneuma, *see* spirit
pneumonia, *see* disease
polio, *see* disease, poliomyelitis
polyethylene glycol (PEG), **150**
polymerization, 79
Pool, Judith, 95
poppy, 16
potassium, 61, 62
precapillary sphincter, 56, 59
pressure, 56, 59, 60–61, 62, 67, 71

partial, 62, 65
Priestley, Joseph, 27
promonocyte, 107, **107**
prophecy, 19
properdin proteins, 108
prostaglandin (PGI-2), 78
protein, 7, 30–31, 37, 38, 40, 50, **60**, 61, 63, 69, 70, 75, 76, 78, 79, 82, 109–10, 111, 112, 113, 116, 123, 125, 126, 131, 135, 136, 144, 152
    complement, **117**
prothrombin, 81, 84, 86, 94
prothrombin activator, 78–79, 81
provirus, 142
Ptolemy I, 20
pseudopod, 103, 104, 105, **105**, 107
pulse, 20
Pythagoras, 129

R
Race, Robert, 48
radiation, 78
    detector, **147**
    therapy, 140–41, **147**
radioactive phosphorus, 139
radioimmunoassay, 147
Rasputin, 92, 93–94
Reagan, Ronald, 39
reagin, 119, 122
Red Badge of Courage, The, 16
red blood cell, 7, 25, 26, 27, 30, **30**, 31, **32**, 33, 37, 38, 39, 40, 46, 47, 48, 50, **64**, 65, 67, 69, 76, 77, 78, **78**, 79, 80, 85, 102, 107, 109, 126, 129, 132, **133**, 135, 136, 137, 139, 141, 153, *see also* blood cell, erythrocyte
red corpuscle, *see* blood cell, erythrocyte, corpuscle
religion, 10
renal artery, *see* artery, renal
renin, 59
reproduction, 31
Rh factor, *see* blood type
Robertson, O. H., 51
Rocky Mountain spotted fever, *see* disease
Rouleaux formation, 33
rubella, *see* disease
rubriblast, 31
Rush, Benjamin, 22
Russell, Morgan, 29

S
sacrament, 10
sacrifice, 14, 15
St. Januarius, 12
Salk, Jonas, 99, 100, 106
salt, 30, 31, 72, 80
salvation, 13
Sanger, Ruth, 48
Scribner, Belding, 137
Secret Book of the Physician, The, 19
seizure, **133**, 135

serotonin, 76, 77
serum, 47, 79, 153
serum hepatitis, *see* disease, hepatitis
Servetus, Miguel, 25
Settle, Dorothy, 132
shock, 52, 81, 153
shroud of Turin, 13
sickle cell anemia, *see* disease, anemia
sickle cell trait, **136, 137**
sickling crisis, 135, 136
Siniscalco, Marcello, 129
sinusoid, 70, **70**, 71
"606", 99
slow-reacting substance of anaphylaxis
    (SRS-A), 125
smallpox, *see* disease
sodium, 61, 62, 136
   citrate, 51
   cyanate, 136–37
solutes, 72
Spaet, Theodore, 77
specific immune system, 108
spermatozoa, 26
spirit, 20
   animal, 20
   natural, 20
   vital, 20
spleen, 31, **83**, 109, 110, 113, 125, 135, 151
Stalin, Joseph, 24
Starling, E. H., 31
stem cell, 110, 125
stomach, 29, 71, 108, **133**
strength, 9, 18
streptokinase, 87–88
striated muscle, **78**
stroke, *see* disease
sugar, 30, 59, 69, 109–10, 112, 113, 125
suppressant, 149
suppressor T cells, 149
surface receptors, 112
surgery, 23, 24
sweat gland, 108
sympathetic healing, 21
sympathetic nervous system, 81
syphilis, *see* disease
systematic lupus erythmatosus (SLE), *see*
   disease, lupus
systemic circulation, *see* circulation
systole, 20

T
Talisman, The, 18
temperament, 17
tetanus, *see* disease

throat, 62, 108
thrombin, 29, 81, 82, 94
thrombocyte, *see* blood cell, platelet
thromboplastin, *see* tissue factor
thrombus, 81–82, 84, 86, 87, 88
thymus gland, 110, 125, 126
tissue, 31, 38, 39, 56, 59, 60, 65, 66, 67, 69,
   70, 78, 79, 81, 104, 107, 108, 109, 115,
   124, **133**, 149
   factor, 78
   histiocyte, 105
   macrophage system, 84
tolerance, 125, 126
tonsil, 109
total-body irradiation, 141
total therapy, 140
toxin, 102, 103, 104, 107, 109
transfusion, 41, 44–46, 47, 49, 52, 95, 119,
   139, 147, 153
transplant, 45
transubstantiation, 12
Trichinella, 41
tuberculosis, *see* disease
tubule, 71, 72
tumor, 142, 144
typhoid fever, *see* disease
typhus, *see* disease

U
urea, **30**, 61, 72
uremia, 72
ureter, 71
urine, 19, 71–72, 87, 147
urokinase, **83**, 87, 88
urushiol, 123

V
vaccination, 97–99, 100, 101, 106, 113,
   120, 136, 147, 149, 152
vaccinia, *see* disease, cowpox
variolation, 98
vascular spasm, 75
vasoconstrictor agent, 60
vasomotor center, 59
vasopressin, 59
vegetable toxin, 129
vein, 15, 19, 20, 27, 43, 45, 47, 56, **57**, 59,
   59, 64, 70, **70**, 71, 81, 82, 87, 88, 108,
   111, 135, 153
   hepatic, **57**, **70**, 71
   jugular, 10, 80
   portal, 25, 70, **70**, 71, 72
   pulmonary, **57**

thoracic, 111, **111**
vena cava, 70, **70**
venesection, 137
venule, 56, 59, **59**, **64**, 70, 107, 120
   pulmonary, 62
Vesalius, Andreas, 25
Victoria, 91, **91**, 92
villus, 69, 70
violence, 17
Virchow, Rudolf, 99
"virgin's disease," *see* disease, anemia
virus, 40, 41, 97, 101, 102, 106, 107, 108,
   109, 113, 115, 116, 120, 135, 139,
   141–42, 147, 149, 151, 152
vitamin, 7, 31
   B$_{12}$, 133, **133**, 135
   K, 84, 86
   deficiency, 84, 88
vitamin deficiency anemia, *see* disease,
   anemia
Vroman, Leo, 31

W
Waller, Augustus Volney, 100
war, 16, 17, 18
waste, 29, 31, 39, 56, 59, 60, 72, 142
water, 55, 69, 70, 71–72
Weinstein, Howard, 141
white blood cell, 7, 30, **30**, **32**, 39, 40, 41,
   48, 76, 82, 84, 97, 100, 102, 103, 104,
   107, 108, 109, 111, 131, 139, 140, 141,
   142, 149, *see also* blood cell, leukocyte
white spot, 39
whooping cough, *see* disease, pertussis
Wiernik, Peter, 141
windpipe, **62**
World War I, 16, 51
wound, 7, 13, 16, 24–25, 52, 75, 76, 78, 79,
   81, 82, 88, 100, 114, 142
Wren, Chistopher, 13
Wright, Almroth, 94
Wright, James Homer, 76

X
X-ray, 141
X-ray crystallography, 50

Y
yellow fever, *see* disease
young blood, 17

Z
zymogens, 78